An Evaluation of Emerging Driver Fatigue Detection Measures and Technologies

Final Report

U.S. Department of Transportation

Federal Motor Carrier Safety Administration

June 2009

FOREWORD

Operator fatigue and sleep deprivation have been widely recognized as critical safety issues that cut across all modes in the transportation industry. FMCSA, the trucking industry, highway safety advocates, and transportation researchers have all identified driver fatigue as a high-priority commercial vehicle safety issue. Fatigue affects mental alertness, decreasing an individual's ability to operate a vehicle safely and increasing the risk of human error that could lead to fatalities and injuries. Sleepiness slows reaction time, decreases awareness, and impairs judgment. Fatigue and sleep deprivation impact all transportation operators (airline pilots, truck drivers, and railroad engineers, for example).

Adding to the difficulty of understanding the fatigue problem and developing effective countermeasures to address operator fatigue is the fact that the incidence of fatigue is underestimated because it is so hard to quantify and measure. Obtaining reliable data on fatigue-related crashes is challenging because it is difficult to determine the degree to which fatigue plays a role in crashes. Fatigue, however, can be managed, and effectively managing fatigue will result in a significant reduction in related risk and improved safety.

This study focuses on recent developments in mathematical models and vehicle-based operator alertness-monitoring technologies. The major objective of this paper is to review and discuss many of the activities currently underway to develop unobtrusive, in-vehicle, real-time drowsy driver detection and fatigue-monitoring/alerting systems.

Although this report can be helpful to the general public in understanding driver fatigue detection measures and technologies, the report is primarily targeted towards commercial motor carrier fleets and their drivers.

This publication is considered a final report and does not supersede another publication.

NOTICE

Technical Report Documentation Page

1. Report No. FMCSA-RRR-09-005	2. Government Accession No.	3. Recipient's Catalog No.
4. Title and Subtitle: **An Evaluation of Emerging Driver Fatigue Detection Measures and Technologies**		5. Report Date: **June 2009**
7. Author(s): **Lawrence Barr, Stephen Popkin, and Heidi Howarth**	6. Performing Organization Code	
	8. Performing Organization Report No.	
9. Performing Organization Name and Address: **Volpe National Transportation Systems Center** **55 Broadway, Kendall Square** **Cambridge, MA 02142**	10. Work Unit No.	
	11. Contract or Grant No. **SA-1J/CB136**	
12. Sponsoring Agency Name and Address: **U.S. Department of Transportation** **Federal Motor Carrier Safety Administration,** **Office of Analysis, Research and Technology** **1200 New Jersey Ave. SE** **Washington, DC 20590**	13. Type of Report and Period Covered **Final Report** **January 2005 – November 2006**	
	14. Sponsoring Agency Code **FMCSA**	
15. Supplementary Notes: **Robert J. Carroll was the FMCSA contracting officer technical representative for this project.**		

16. Abstract:

Operator fatigue and sleep deprivation have been widely recognized as critical safety issues that cut across all modes in the transportation industry. FMCSA, the trucking industry, highway safety advocates, and transportation researchers have all identified driver fatigue as a high priority commercial vehicle safety issue. Fatigue affects mental alertness, decreasing an individual's ability to operate a vehicle safely and increasing the risk of human error that could lead to fatalities and injuries. Sleepiness slows reaction time, decreases awareness, and impairs judgment. Fatigue and sleep deprivation impact all transportation operators (airline pilots, truck drivers, and railroad engineers, for example).

Adding to the difficulty of understanding the fatigue problem and developing effective countermeasures to address operator fatigue is the fact that the incidence of fatigue is underestimated because it is so hard to quantify and measure. Obtaining reliable data on fatigue-related crashes is challenging because it is difficult to determine the degree to which fatigue plays a role in crashes. Fatigue, however, can be managed, and effectively managing fatigue will result in a significant reduction in related risk and improved safety.

This study focuses on recent developments in mathematical models and vehicle-based operator alertness monitoring technologies. The major objective of this paper is to review and discuss many of the activities currently underway to develop unobtrusive, in-vehicle, real-time drowsy driver detection and fatigue-monitoring/alerting systems.

17. Key Words: **Alertness, Circadian, Commercial Motor Vehicle, Driver, Drowsiness, Fatigue, Highway Safety, Sleepiness, Truck**		18. Distribution Statement	
19. Security Classif. (of this report) **Unclassified**	20. Security Classif. (of this page) **Unclassified**	21. No. of Pages: **55**	22. Price **N/A**

Form DOT F 1700.7 (8-72) Reproduction of completed page authorized.

SI* (MODERN METRIC) CONVERSION FACTORS

APPROXIMATE CONVERSIONS TO SI UNITS

Symbol	When You Know	Multiply By	To Find	Symbol
		LENGTH		
in	inches	25.4	millimeters	mm
ft	feet	0.305	meters	m
yd	yards	0.914	meters	m
mi	miles	1.61	kilometers	km
		AREA		
in^2	square inches	645.2	square millimeters	mm^2
ft^2	square feet	0.093	square meters	m^2
yd^2	square yards	0.836	square meters	m^2
ac	acres	0.405	hectares	ha
mi^2	square miles	2.59	square kilometers	km^2
		VOLUME		
fl oz	fluid ounces	29.57	milliliters	ml
gal	gallons	3.785	liters	l
ft^3	cubic feet	0.028	cubic meters	m^3
yd^3	cubic yards	0.765	cubic meters	m^3
		MASS		
oz	ounces	28.35	grams	g
lb	pounds	0.454	kilograms	kg
T	short tons (2000 lbs)	0.907	megagrams	Mg
		TEMPERATURE (exact)		
°F	Fahrenheit temperature	5(F-32)/9 or (F-32)/1.8	Celsius temperature	°C
		ILLUMINATION		
fc	foot-candles	10.76	lux	lx
fl	foot-Lamberts	3.426	candela/m2	cd/m2
		FORCE and PRESSURE or STRESS		
lbf	pound-force	4.45	newtons	N
psi	pound-force per square inch	6.89	kilopascals	kPa

APPROXIMATE CONVERSIONS FROM SI UNITS

Symbol	When You Know	Multiply By	To Find	Symbol
		LENGTH		
mm	millimeters	0.039	inches	in
m	meters	3.28	feet	ft
m	meters	1.09	Yards	yd
km	kilometers	0.621	miles	mi
		AREA		
mm^2	square millimeters	0.0016	square inches	in^2
m^2	square meters	10.764	square feet	ft^2
m^2	square meters	1.195	square yards	yd^2
ha	hectares	2.47	acres	ac
km^2	square kilometers	0.386	square miles	mi^2
		VOLUME		
ml	milliliters	0.034	fluid ounces	fl oz
l	liters	0.264	gallons	gal
m^3	cubic meters	35.71	cubic feet	ft^3
m^3	cubic meters	1.307	cubic yards	yd^3
		MASS		
g	grams	0.035	ounces	oz
kg	kilograms	2.202	pounds	lb
Mg	megagrams	1.103	short tons (2000 lbs)	T
		TEMPERATURE (exact)		
°C	Celsius temperature	1.8 C + 32	Fahrenheit temperature	°F
		ILLUMINATION		
lx	lux	0.0929	foot-candles	fc
cd/m2	candela/m2	0.2919	foot-Lamberts	fl
		FORCE and PRESSURE or STRESS		
N	newtons	0.225	pound-force	lbf
kPa	kilopascals	0.145	pound-force per square inch	psi

* SI is the symbol for the International System of Units. Appropriate rounding should be made to comply with Section 4 of ASTM E380.

TABLE OF CONTENTS

LIST OF TABLES

LIST OF FIGURES

LIST OF ACRONYMS

AECS	Average Eye Closure Speed
ANN	Artificial Neural Network
APL	Applied Physics laboratory
ASL	Applied Science Laboratories
ASTiD	Advisory System for Tired Drives
AVR Am	plitude-velocity ratio
BLINKD Eye-blink	duration
CAS	Circadian Alertness Simulator model
DDDS	Drowsy Driver Detection System
DFM	Driver Fatigue Monitor
DSM Driver	State Monitor
EEG Electroencephalography	
EU European	Union
FAID Fatigue	Audit InterDyne model
FMCSA	Federal Motor Carrier Safety Administration
FOT	Field operational test
GWU	George Washington University
IR Infrared	
KSS Karolinska	Sleepiness Scale
LED Light-em	itting diode
NHTSA	National Highway Traffic Safety Administration
R&D	Research and Development
RPI	Rensselaer Polytechnic Institute
SAFE	System of Aircrew Fatigue Evaluation model
SAFTE	Sleep, Activity, Fatigue and Task Effectiveness model
SDLAT Standard	deviation of lateral position
SEFO Sensor	foil
SENSATION	Advanced Sensor Development for Attention, Stress, Vigilance and Sleep/Wakefulness Monitoring
TOVA	Test of Variables Attention
USDOT	U.S. Department of Transportation

EXECUTIVE SUMMARY

The primary mission of the Federal Motor Carrier Safety Administration (FMCSA) of the U.S. Department of Transportation (USDOT) is to promote the safety of commercial motor vehicle transportation and to prevent commercial vehicle-related fatalities and injuries. An important element in meeting FMCSA's strategic safety objectives is an emphasis on the safety performance of commercial drivers to ensure they are physically qualified to operate commercial motor vehicles safely while staying mentally alert. The authors completed a survey study to identify, review, and evaluate emerging driver alertness detection measures, models, and technologies that can be used to provide 24-hour fatigue monitoring capability.

Operator fatigue and sleep deprivation have been widely recognized as critical safety issues that cut across all modes in the transportation industry. FMCSA, the trucking industry, highway safety advocates, and transportation researchers have all identified driver fatigue as a high-priority commercial vehicle safety issue. Fatigue affects mental alertness, decreasing an individual's ability to operate a vehicle safely and increasing the risk of human error that could lead to fatalities and injuries. Sleepiness slows reaction time, decreases awareness, and impairs judgment. Fatigue and sleep deprivation impact all transportation operators (such as airline pilots, truck drivers, and railroad engineers) (Sullivan 2003).

Adding to the difficulty of understanding the fatigue problem and developing effective countermeasures to address operator fatigue is the fact that the incidence of fatigue is underestimated because it is so hard to quantify and measure. Obtaining reliable data on fatigue-related crashes is challenging because it is difficult to determine the degree to which fatigue plays a role in crashes. For instance, if a motorist is unharmed in a crash, the resulting increased arousal following the incident usually masks the impairment that could assist investigating officers in attributing the crash to drowsiness. As a result, sleepiness as a contributing factor in motor vehicle crashes is underreported in crash databases that are based on police accident reports. Moreover, because sleep deprivation increases the likelihood of attention lapses, drowsiness or fatigue may play a role in crashes attributed to other causes as well. An investigator may report that a crash was caused by a driver running a red light, whereas in reality the crash occurred because the driver was not appropriately vigilant due to his or her state of sleepiness and fatigue (Sullivan 2003). And finally, drivers tend to be poor judges of their own level of drowsiness; that is, they cannot reliably predict when they are impaired to the point of falling asleep at the wheel.

In addition to the lack of available data and the problem of underestimation, Rosekind (1998) identifies three formidable challenges in successfully addressing the issue of fatigue in the commercial motor vehicle industry. First of all, operational requirements are diverse; that is, the trucking industry incorporates a wide range of driving requirements. Factors such as work schedules, duty times, rest periods, recovery opportunities, and respoU to customer needs can vary widely. Second, there are considerable individual differences among operators. For example, age can have a significant effect on the quality and quantity of sleep an individual might obtain or need, on a person's ability to cope with rotating shift schedules or night work, and on the risk for sleep disorders. And finally, the interaction of the principal physiological factors that underlie fatigue, namely the homeostatic drive for sleep and circadian rhythms, is a complex issue. These challenges preclude a single, simple solution to the fatigue problem and suggest that it may be impractical to expect that fatigue can be completely eliminated from 24-hour transportation operations. Fatigue can, however, be managed, and effectively managing fatigue will result in a significant reduction in related risk and improved safety (Rosekind 1998).

Successfully reducing fatigue-related risks in transportation will require some innovative concepts and evolving approaches. Available and emerging technology approaches have great potential as a relevant and effective tool to address fatigue. Dinges and Mallis (1998) described the following four categories of operator-centered alertness monitoring and fatigue detection and prediction technologies:

1. **Readiness-to-perform and fitness-for-duty technologies.** These systems attempt to assess reaction time, psychomotor tracking, or vigilance and alertness capacity of an operator before the work is performed (i.e., prior to the start of the work shift). The primary objective of fitness-for-duty tests is to establish whether the operator is fit by evaluating his/her functional work capability at the start of a given work shift and the ability to work through the duration of the entire duty period. These tests generally fall into one of two groups: performance-based tests (e.g., measuring reaction time) or tests that measure ocular physiology (Krueger 2004; Hartley et al. 2000).

2. **Mathematical models/algorithm technologies.** This approach involves the application of mathematical models that predict operator alertness and performance at different times, based on interactions of the amount of sleep obtained or missed, on circadian factors, on the present workload, and on related temporal antecedents of fatigue (Dinges and Mallis 1998; Dinges 1997). These highly complex algorithms allow for individual patterns of sleep, work, and rest to be entered into a system that will then produce outputs describing how levels of performance will be affected by the individual's sleep/work history. These models make up the subclass of operator-centered technologies that includes those devices that seek to monitor sources of fatigue, such as how much sleep an operator has obtained, and combine this information with a mathematical model designed to predict performance capability over a period of time and to predict when future periods of increased sleepiness will occur (Dinges and Mallis 1998; Krueger 2004; Hartley et al. 2000).

3. **Vehicle-based performance technologies.** These technologies mainly include those that measure vehicle performance parameters (e.g., steering movements, vehicle speed, or the movements of the vehicle within the lane markers on the roadway), and they infer driver behavior by monitoring the continuity of steering wheel movements and/or vehicle speed, or by examining the driver's ability to maintain adequate lane-tracking movements while steering the vehicle (Hartley et al. 2000). Vehicle-based performance technologies have a sound basis in research, which revealed that vehicle control and driver performance are impaired by fatigue. These technologies generally involve no intrusive monitoring devices, and the output relates to the actual performance of the driver controlling the vehicle (Krueger 2004).

4. **Vehicle-based operator alertness/drowsiness/vigilance monitoring technologies.** These technologies exemplify the most common approaches currently used to monitor driver fatigue, and they monitor—usually on-line and in real time—some biobehavioral aspect of the operator such as eye gaze, eye closure, pupil occlusion, head position and movement, brain wave activity, heart rate, etc. To be practical and useful as a driver

assistance system, these devices must acquire, interpret, and feed back information in real-world driving environments. There is a tremendous need to demonstrate the efficacy of operator-based on-board fatigue monitoring technologies in a real-world naturalistic driving environment, and a significant amount of effort is ongoing in this area.

This study focuses on recent developments in mathematical models and vehicle-based operator alertness monitoring technologies. The major objective of this paper is to review and discuss many of the activities currently underway to develop unobtrusive, in-vehicle, real-time drowsy driver detection and fatigue-monitoring/alerting systems. An on-board device that monitors a driver's level of fatigue and drowsiness in real time is an important component of a comprehensive and effective fatigue management program. People suffering from fatigue exhibit certain behaviors that are easily observable from facial features such as the eyelid closures. Observable behaviors that typically reflect a person's level of fatigue include eyelid, pupil, and head movement, as well as facial expression (Ji et al. 2004). To make use of these observable cues of sleepiness, a considerable amount of research is currently aimed at developing noninvasive techniques for assessing a driver's alertness level through the visual observation of his/her physical condition using a remote camera and state-of-the-art technologies in computer vision. Recent progress in machine vision research and advances in computer hardware technologies have made it possible to measure head pose, eye gaze, and eyelid movement with a high degree of accuracy using video cameras. In a conference sponsored by the U.S. Department of Transportation on ocular measures of driver alertness, Wierwille (1999) identified computer vision as the most promising noninvasive technology for monitoring driver alertness. This report also provides a review of several biomathematical models of human fatigue and performance that have been developed and commercialized in recent years.

In the following section, the key features of several mathematical models that have been developed to predict operator alertness and performance are summarized. Next, the general design guidelines for a practical in-vehicle fatigue detection and monitoring system are outlined in Section 3. An overview of several promising technologies that are currently in use or that will be available in the near future is presented in Section 4. Some of the important technical features and operational characteristics are described in this section, as well as a brief summary of the development status for each of the systems. In addition, a methodological framework is offered for assessing the user interface needs and acceptance criteria of truck operators and fatigue managers for on-board alertness detection and monitoring technologies. And finally, Section 5 highlights several emerging technologies that were presented in an international conference in Basel, Switzerland in May 2006.

1. MATHEMATICAL MODELS OF FATIGUE AND PERFORMANCE

Biomathematical models that quantify the effects of circadian and sleep/wake processes on the regulation of alertness and performance have been developed in an effort to predict the magnitude and timing of fatigue-related respoUs in transportation operations (Dinges et al. 2004). These models of fatigue and performance typically use input information about sleep history, duration of wakefulness, work and rest patterns, and circadian phase to predict sleepiness, performance capability, and/or fatigue risk. They are being applied to assess vulnerability to fatigue and performance degradation as a function of time of day, to design and evaluate work/rest schedules, to plan work and sleep in operational missions, to assist in determining the timing of countermeasures to anticipated performance deficits, and for accident assessment and policy-making (e.g., hours-of-service regulations).

In respoU to the escalating interest in biomathematical models to predict operator alertness and performance, and also given the rapid development and commercialization of these models, a workshop was held in 2002 to examine and review the state-of-the-art fatigue and performance models. This section summarizes and describes the key features of seven biomathematical models that have been recently developed and/or made commercially available. These models were presented at the 2002 Fatigue and Performance Modeling Workshop.

1.1 TWO-PROCESS MODEL

The two-process model of sleep regulation (Borbely 1982) is at the core of many biomathematical models that address the regulation of fatigue and performance. The model is based on the interaction of its two constituent processes, the homeostatic Process S and the circadian Process C, which generate the timing of sleep and waking. It assumes that the level of the sleep/wake-dependent Process S rises during waking and declines during sleep, and that it interacts with a circadian Process C. In addition to the timing of sleep, changes of daytime vigilance are accounted for by the interaction of the homeostatic and circadian processes.

The two-process model has inspired a considerable number of experiments and stimulated the establishment of other models of neurobehavioral functions. The attractiveness of the approach is due to its physiological appeal and its mathematical simplicity. The model allows the simulation of the timing of both sleep and wakefulness and sleepiness and alertness. It was created using laboratory data from a number of experiments, including power spectral analysis of electroencephalographic (EEG) slow wave activity during non-REM sleep. Model validity has been demonstrated in successful simulations under various sleep conditions (Achermann 2004).

1.2 SLEEP/WAKE PREDICTOR MODEL

The Sleep/Wake Predictor Model (Akerstedt et al. 2004), also referred to as the Three-Process Model of Alertness, is a computer model that uses the timing of work and/or sleep hours as input and uses both a circadian and a homeostatic component (amount of prior wake and amount of prior sleep) to predict subjective alertness and performance in daily life. The purpose of the Sleep/Wake Predictor Model is to provide the following:

- An integrated and quantitative description of the main factors that affect alertness and alertness-related performance
- A method for predicting alertness from knowledge of sleep/wake patterns or only work patterns
- Quantitative support for evaluation of work/rest schedules in terms of alertness, fatigue, performance impairment, and accident risk
- A quantitative tool for monitoring the state of alertness and fatigue-related error risk
- An educational tool for teaching sleep/wake regulation and fatigue consciousness
- A tool for generating research hypotheses regarding sleep/wake regulation and its coUquences

Using subjective alertness data from a number of experiments of altered sleep/wake patterns, the model predicts alertness on the basis of four parameters or components: S, C, W, and U. Process S is an exponential function representing the time since awakening, and the model assumes an exponential drop in alertness during the waking period and an exponential rise in alertness after sleep. Process C represents sleepiness due to circadian influences and has a sinusoidal form with an afternoon peak at approximately 5:00 p.m. Process W is an exponential sleep inertia factor that simulates the wakeup process. The final component in the model is Process U, for "ultradian," that simulates the afternoon dip in alertness. No assumptions are made other than that of a normal eight-hour sleep when starting the simulation.

The target markets identified for use of the Sleep/Wake Predictor Model include researchers in sleep/wake regulation and in shift work; occupational specialists and hygienists who need information on human physiology and performance in relation to work hours; government organizations in charge of safety, health, and work-hour regulations; and company schedulers and planning staff who want to evaluate the fatigue and performance effects of particular work schedules, such as those used by the road, sea, air, and rail transport sectors. The model software interface provides screen output including sleep variables (latency, duration, bedtime), alertness and performance curves, accident risk, as well as printer file outputs for all curves and start and end times of all sleep periods.

1.3   SYSTEM FOR AIRCREW FATIGUE EVALUATION MODEL

The System for Aircrew Fatigue Evaluation (SAFE) Model was developed primarily for use in aviation operations based on laboratory experiments and was subsequently adjusted using data collected during actual long-haul flights (Belyavin and Spencer 2004). In its initial form, the model was based on a series of laboratory experiments that investigated the effects of irregular patterns of work and rest on performance during conditions of partial isolation. The experiments were specifically designed to provide irregular patterns of work and rest that avoided overall sleep deprivation. In addition, they permitted efficient estimates to be made of changes in performance at different times of day, during work periods of varying duration. Subjective assessments of alertness were obtained by monitoring performance on the Digit Symbol Substitution Task (among other tasks) at two-hour intervals throughout the waking periods. The model consists of two components, one related to the circadian rhythm and the other to the sleep/wake process.

A significant amount of work has been done to collect information on aircrew fatigue and levels of alertness in flight so that the model could be confidently applied to air operations. The diary, questionnaire, and sleep log studies that were completed helped to identify factors relevant to aviation operations that influence the subjective levels of alertness, in addition to those defined in the basic model. These have been incorporated into the latest version of SAFE, and include the following:

- Multiple sectors—A factor related to the number of flights undertaken within a given duty period

- Time on task—A factor related to the duration of the duty period

- Cumulative fatigue—A factor representing a decline in alertness associated with coUcutive duties and with the build-up in fatigue over long tours of duty

- Early starts—A model correction to allow for reduced levels of alertness throughout duty periods starting before 9:00 a.m.

- Daytime sleep—A factor to reduce the amount of recuperation provided by sleep taken outside the normal nighttime period or at unusual times

- In-flight rest—An algorithm to predict the duration of in-flight sleep as a function of the timing and duration of the rest period (i.e., the time that the pilot is away from the controls)

Results of the model are displayed graphically in two-week time frames, and estimates of sleep times are an optional display. Alertness levels during duty periods are presented on a color-coded display.

1.4   INTERACTIVE NEUROBEHAVIORAL MODEL

The Interactive Neurobehavioral Model estimates neurobehavioral performance, which is determined by a linear combination of circadian, homeostatic, and sleep inertia components. Development of the model was targeted for scientific researchers; the National Aeronautics and Space Administration; Department of DefeU schedulers; shift/duty schedulers in the trucking, aviation, and railway industries; and agencies that regulate duty hours, such as the Federal Aviation Administration. The model's software works on a PC and allows the user to input both light levels and sleep/wake times for the specific schedule to be simulated. Text output files, which can be read in any graphical program, are generated to predict performance and alertness levels and minimum core body temperature. In addition, the software is able to generate graphs of the input protocol and output results (Dinges et al. 2004).

Validation assessments of the Interactive Neurobehavioral Model have been performed by comparing model predictions with neurobehavioral data collected in laboratory studies of human subjects involving varying light patterns, simulated jet lag, sleep deprivation, and non-24 hour schedules.

1.5   SLEEP, ACTIVITY, FATIGUE, AND TASK EFFECTIVENESS MODEL

The Sleep, Activity, Fatigue, and Task Effectiveness (SAFTE) Model was developed for use in both military and industrial settings, and current users include the U.S. Air Force and the Federal Railroad Administration (Balkin et al. 2004). The model has been applied to the construction of a Fatigue Avoidance Scheduling Tool (Eddy and Hursh 2001), which is designed to help optimize the operational management of aviation ground and flight crews, but is not limited to this application.

The fundamental structure of the SAFTE Model incorporates the three recognized components that influence neurobehavioral performance and that are included in most models: homeostatic, circadian, and sleep inertia. Overall "effectiveness" is a linear sum of these three components. Sleep times and duration are generated based on either real-world data or an "auto sleep" algorithm. The model assumes that sleep occurs between 10:00 p.m. and 6:00 a.m.; however, these times can be adjusted in the software interface to represent actual sleep schedules. The software interface provides the schedule input and predictions (e.g., cognitive and physical performance) in graphical and tabular form, parameter tables used for adjusting the model, and description boxes for schedules and events. The primary model output is performance effectiveness.

The current version of the model is based on data collected on college-age students during laboratory studies. The model has been validated against literature studies and laboratory-conducted sleep deprivation research, and future plans include validation against actual performance of railroad engineers. Currently the SAFTE Model does not include the effects of physical work, workload, or level of interest in task. Two additional limitations are that the model does not provide an estimate of group variance about the average performance prediction and it does not incorporate any individual difference parameters, such as age, chronotype (morningness/eveningness), and individual sleep requirements.

1.6   FATIGUE AUDIT INTERDYNE MODEL

The Fatigue Audit InterDyne (FAID) Model (Dawson et al. 2004) can be used to quantify the work-related fatigue associated with any duty schedule using hours of work (i.e., start/end times of work periods) as the sole input. The researchers who developed FAID believe that models requiring actual or estimated sleep times as one of several inputs pose difficulties for organizations that want to estimate the effects of fatigue in workplace settings (as opposed to laboratory-based studies). In work-related situations, reliance on actual sleep times as a model input is problematic because it is difficult, costly, and time-consuming to collect objective measures of sleep/wake times for every possible duty schedule. Also, reliance of estimated sleep times as an input is problematic because it requires subjective judgment. Hence, a major advantage of FAID is that it does not require actual or estimated sleep/wake records as an input. Rather, it assigns a "recovery value" to time away from work based on the amount of sleep that is likely to be obtained in non-work periods, depending on the length of those periods and the time of day that they occur.

In FAID, a duty schedule is viewed as a time-varying function whereby an individual is considered to be either working or not working. The model is based on the conceptual notion that the fatigue level associated with a duty schedule is determined by a balance between fatigue accumulated during work periods and the amount of recovery obtained during non-work periods. The fatigue levels of work periods and the recovery values of rest periods are dependent upon their length, circadian timing, and "recency" over the seven-day preceding work history. Essentially, longer work periods are more fatiguing than shorter work periods, and nighttime work periods are more fatiguing than daytime work periods. In addition, the fatigue values of work periods and the recovery values of non-work periods are weighted such that more recent work and non-work periods make a greater relative contribution to the overall fatigue score than less recent periods.

In summary, the FAID Model was created from existing research collected during controlled laboratory experiments on the performance-diminishing effects of wakefulness and the restorative effects of sleep. It was developed to be used in workplace settings to quantify the work-related fatigue associated with past, current, and proposed duty schedules. Since the model uses hours of work as the only input parameter, it enables estimates of the work-related fatigue associated with any duty schedule to be made using information that is readily available in schedule and/or payroll records. Additional research efforts are being applied to provide further validation of FAID in laboratory, simulator, and workplace settings and to modify the model to improve its predictive power.

1.7   CIRCADIAN ALERTNESS SIMULATOR MODEL

The Circadian Alertness Simulator (CAS) Model was developed by Circadian Technologies, Inc. as a practical tool for assessing the risk of diminished alertness in the workplace and for reducing the rate of fatigue-related accidents, injuries, and fatalities at work. Applications include work schedule optimization, fatigue-related accident investigation, and employee lifestyle education training. CAS has been used as a fatigue assessment system in several fatigue management projects in the railroad and trucking industries, and it has been proven to be an effective tool in employee fatigue reduction programs (Aguirre et al. 2004).

CAS uses actual work patterns to simulate chronic fatigue levels. Based on the documented work schedules of employees, sleep and alertness patterns are estimated and a cumulative fatigue risk score is calculated across multiple days or weeks. The current version of CAS is tailored for irregular work schedules in the transportation industry. Future versions of the model will include regular rotating schedules and jetlag applications consisting of travel across time zones.

The CAS Model is based on the two-process model of sleep regulation (Borbely 1982), where sleep timing and duration are determined by the relationships between circadian factors (phase, period, amplitude), homeostatic components (sleep and wake duration), and alertness. In the CAS Model, the circadian component is assumed to have a sinusoidal function with a 24-hour period. The homeostatic component is assumed to have an exponential increase during sleep and an exponential decrease during wakefulness; that is, it recognizes that recuperation is more rapid in the initial hours of sleep and that loss of alertness is more rapid during the initial hours of wakefulness, with the growth of alertness limited by an upper threshold.

For the majority of applications in which the precise hours of sleep and wakefulness are not known, the CAS software creates an estimated sleep/wake pattern based on the actual work pattern of the individual. In cases where actual data on sleep/wake patterns are available, these data can be entered directly into the model and the sleep estimation algorithm is bypassed. Using either simulated or actual sleep, a continuous alertness curve ranging from 0 (low alertness) to 100 (high alertness) is computed. In default mode, the CAS software simulates sleep and alertness for an average individual; however, the model settings can be adjusted to simulate data for specific individual characteristics such as chronotype (morningness/eveningness), habitual wakeup time, habitual sleep length, napping capability, or sleep flexibility. Finally, a cumulative fatigue score is calculated for each individual or group of individuals based on sleep measures and the actual work/rest pattern. The fatigue score ranges from 0 (no fatigue) to 100 (extreme fatigue). It quantifies overall fatigue risk across a given period and is intended to be applied as a measure for assessment of operational fatigue.

To test and demonstrate the validity of CAS, it was applied to compute fatigue risk using the work/rest and accident data from three trucking operations. Specifically, the cumulative fatigue score was used as a metric to help reduce fatigue-related accident risk. The model developers reported that the use of such a fatigue risk assessment tool significantly reduced the rate and severity of heavy-truck accidents. Also, truck drivers involved in DOT-recordable or high-cost crashes were found to have significantly higher CAS fatigue risk scores than accident-free drivers.

In summary, Circadian Technologies states that CAS meets the following three criteria necessary for a mathematical model of fatigue to be operationally useful: (1) It combines the complex interactions between factors such as length of shift, time of day, sequence of shift rotations, number of coUcutive work days, and other factors that influence employee fatigue into a single fatigue risk score on which day-to-day work scheduling and overtime assignment decisions can be made; (2) it demonstrates a correlation between the fatigue risk score calculated by the model and the rate of fatigue-related accidents in the workplace; and (3) it provides evidence that employee work/rest scheduling decisions made by managers using the model can result in a reduction in accident rate and costs.

2. TECHNICAL AND DESIGN GUIDELINES

The guidelines and criteria used to assess the potential efficacy of the candidate alertness monitoring technologies and devices relate to the functional characteristics and operational properties of the device or technology. In most cases, this list lacks the technical details necessary to be considered a functional requirements specification. Nevertheless, addressing user acceptance by employing a structured assessment methodology and evaluating devices against scientific criteria is vital to ensure that any proposed device or technology is qualified for its intended purpose of monitoring, unobtrusively and in real time, driver alertness and thereby potentially helping to mitigate motor vehicle crashes related to driver drowsiness. A list of possible implementation issues is also presented.

2.1   USER ACCEPTANCE ASSESSMENT METHODOLOGY

Regardless of the projected safety benefit for any given vehicle drowsy detection technology, successful deployment is unlikely if users do not deem the device acceptable. Past work in this area (Dinges and Mallis 1998; Whitlock 2002; and Bekiaris et al. 2004a) has specified a number of criteria that should be considered when evaluating the user acceptance of such technologies. Building on these efforts where practical, DOT has conceptualized a methodology to systematically assess user acceptance for the purposes of the evaluation of various new and emerging vehicle technologies. This methodology is largely based on the *NHTSA ITS Strategic Plan for 1997–2002* (NHTSA 1997) and has evolved and been expanded iteratively for USDOT projects involving field operational tests (FOTs) (e.g., Boyle et al. 2001; Barr et al. 2002). In this approach, acceptance is dependent upon the degree to which a driver perceives the benefits derived from a system as being greater than the costs. If a system's potential for safety is not perceived to outweigh its costs, it is likely that the system will not be purchased, or will be purchased but not utilized. Conversely, if device use is perceived to enhance safety potential and driving skill, then there is a chance that those users will feel comfortable engaging in riskier-than-usual driving behavior or otherwise become over-reliant on the system. For a complete evaluation of the safety and user acceptance of such technologies, it is important that each of these outcomes be assessed.

The assessment methodology was developed by deconstructing user acceptance into five broad conceptual elements: *ease of use, ease of learning, perceived value, driver behavior,* and *advocacy*. Systematic evaluation of these elements requires collecting a variety of data in order to address multiple criteria, each of which is based on human factors principles as applied to such technologies. Data sources may include objective measures of performance (MOP), such as those related to driving performance, as well as subjective measures, such as surveys to assess driver attitudes pre- and post-device exposure. Although laboratory and bench testing may be useful in the initial design and evaluation stages, in order to fully address user acceptance and obtain useful and representative data, longitudinal field-testing of safety technologies is ultimately necessary.

Field operational tests offer the benefits of a naturalistic driving setting and the ability to assess usage and acceptance over time, given prolonged exposure to the technology. As part of developing an experimental design, statistical power and effect size should be assessed a priori. Additionally, multiple weeks of data collection for both control and experimental driver groups, as well as baseline and device exposure conditions, are typically required. Subsequent analysis of the objective FOT data, combined with survey analysis to substantiate driver attitudes, integrates multiple data sources with the goal of convergent support for the user acceptance of a device.

Table 1 depicts the user acceptance elements as part of a framework, listing underneath each the related criteria for evaluation. As indicated above, the five user acceptance elements are ease of use, ease of learning, perceived value, driver behavior, and advocacy. These elements and criteria are further described in the text that follows the table, but will likely need to be tailored to the functionality of a specific device, as well as the particular goals of the FOT, when used.

Table 1. Framework of User Acceptance Elements and Criteria for the Evaluation of New and Emerging Vehicle Technologies

Ease of Use	Ease of Learning	Perceived Value	Driver Behavior	Advocacy
Design & usability of device controls	Utility of instructions/ training	Alertness & alertness management enhancement	Control inputs	Willingness to endorse
Use patterns	Ability to retain knowledge of device use	Driving skill enhancement	Awareness/ behavioral adaptation	Purchase interest/intent
Understanding of device state	Time to learn	Safety	Driving style	
Driver accommodation/ variations in information processing		Health concerns	Lifestyle	
Demands on driver/ channel capacity		Confidentiality concerns		
Understanding of warnings/ discriminability of alerts				
Tolerance of false or nuisance warnings				

Ease of use encompasses the degree to which drivers find a technology understandable, usable, and intuitive in its operation and maintenance. Full consideration should be given to the human factors design, usability, and maintenance of a device. Testing may initially take place in a laboratory setting to ensure the accommodation of inherent variability in driver anthropometry and cognitive and physical capabilities, as well as proper operation within various driving environments. Further design and usability evaluation in the field and longitudinally will aid in refining the functionality of such technologies and assessing driver device use patterns over time. Additionally, given various device states, it is critical to determine the degree to which drivers understand the capabilities and limitations of a system, its operational parameters, and what driver actions are expected in assorted situations.

The degree to which a device accommodates individual drivers (i.e., individual differences in perceptual, information processing, physical, and cognitive skills) by promoting correct interpretation of their output must also be evaluated. This includes assessing the demands of attending to the output of an in-vehicle device; a safety technology should not contribute to driver stress or workload. As device feedback typically takes the form of an auditory warning or alert, it is vital that various outputs are easily comprehended, discriminated, and do not conflict with those provided by other safety technologies. Finally, in order to facilitate trust in the safety benefit of such devices, it is crucial that false and/or nuisance alarms are minimized, while maximizing "hits" (i.e., correct assessments of driver status).

Ease of learning as a part of evaluating user acceptance seeks information regarding how well a device is utilized in its intended manner, as well as what is done with such acquired knowledge over time. If a device is well designed, then its operation should be congruent with a user's mental model and therefore easily understood, recalled, and retained. Furthermore, device output should be both intuitive and easily comprehended. Basic testing of such parameters may be conducted in a simulated setting for the evaluation of short-term outcomes. However, only a longitudinal study in field conditions allows for the assessment of learning and unintended device usage. User understanding of the applications of device feedback, both reactively and proactively, in the case of fatigue management planning, is critical for the success of such technologies.

The *perceived value* element of user acceptance assesses the degree to which drivers perceive a safer and/or more alert driving environment as a function of device use. Ideally, the driver is able to utilize such safety-enhancing technologies to facilitate alert vehicle operation, in conjunction with successfully integrating device feedback more broadly into a personal fatigue management program. An additional aspect of perceived value is the degree to which drivers report that these innovations enhance driving performance and safety on the road. When assessing these criteria, it is important to consider the undesirable outcome of drivers' inadvertent or purposeful over-reliance on such technologies to maintain alert and safe vehicle operation. Perceived value may also be impacted to the extent that drivers understand and are informed about device functioning and what aspects of driver behavior the device monitors. For example, if real or perceived health risks are associated with the technology, drivers will weigh such costs against other perceived benefits. Additionally, users may be concerned about data confidentiality to the extent that devices are used to monitor, store, and possibly transmit information regarding their driving behavior.

Alterations in *driver behavior* may occur as a function of device usage over time. Ideally, these changes are intended, positive, and have a permanent impact on safe vehicle operation and driver lifestyle. Evaluating a driver's allocation of cognitive and temporal resources to maintain safe driving serves to ensure that driving behavior is not negatively affected by devices requiring excessive time and cognitive resources to monitor and react to. Additionally, it is important to assess the degree to which driver awareness of and exposure to device feedback over time yields behavioral adaptation. Examples include the extent to which device output is integrated into driving behavior and the potential benefits and/or risks of using a technology in an unintended manner. Further, user acceptance should focus on alterations in driving style (i.e., habits, patterns) that are brought about by modifications to sleep/wake patterns as a result of responding to device output. More broadly, it is important to assess whether extended exposure to such safety devices leads to overall lifestyle changes with regard to fatigue management.

Advocacy is measured in terms of the extent to which drivers consider endorsing or purchasing a safety device, and it is a critical and final component of user acceptance. Ultimately, regardless of a potential safety benefit, and even in spite of perceived benefits on the part of the driver, if a technology is not attainable by the intended users, it will not succeed in the marketplace. Therefore, the willingness of drivers both to purchase a safety device (whether on an individual or commercial basis) and to endorse it to others is a vital aspect of successful deployment.

Where possible, data collection should be planned to include specific objective and subjective measures that individually address and map to each criterion and user acceptance element as outlined above. The criteria used to evaluate the technologies presented in this paper were based on the work of Dinges and Mallis (1996), Whitlock (2002), and Bekiaris et al. (2004a). Ultimately, acceptance attitudes are determined based on the outcomes of statistical analyses that address each of the tailored and specific criteria, as related to stated research objectives.

2.2   SCIENTIFIC/ENGINEERING GUIDELINES

- The device should measure what it is supposed to, operationally (e.g., eye blinks, heart rate, etc.). The device should also measure what its manufacturer purports to measure, conceptually. For example, a device that claims to measure alertness should provide comprehensive evidence of the relationship between the measured variable (e.g., PERCLOS, EEG) and the purported variable (alertness).

- The device should monitor driver behavior in real time.

- The device should be consistent in its measurement over time, and it should measure the same event (operationally and conceptually) for all drivers.

- The device should be able to operate accurately and reliably in both daytime and nighttime illumination conditions.

- For devices that produce audible warnings, it should be possible to hear the auditory output under all driving conditions at a level that is not startling to the user. The volume of auditory output should be adjustable over a reasonable range, approximately 50dB to 90dB.

- The device should be able to operate accurately and reliably in the expected truck cab vibration environment.

- The device should be able to operate over the expected range of truck cab temperature and humidity conditions, in both air-conditioned and non-air-conditioned environments.

- The device should be designed to maximize sensitivity and specificity. In other words, it should accurately and reliably detect reduced alertness when it is actually present (i.e., minimize missed events or false negatives), and it should accurately and reliably identify safe driving and operator vigilance when it is actually present (i.e., minimize false alarms or false positives).

- The device should be able to operate continually and robustly over time with only normal maintenance and replacement costs.

2.3 IMPLEMENTATION ISSUES TO CONSIDER

In addition to the functional criteria listed above, a number of implementation issues should be considered. These issues are not necessarily regarded as requirements against which candidate devices are evaluated, but they are important considerations in the successful implementation and practical use of a device. The user implementation issues include:

- The ergonomics implications of device control and display design and location are critical. The system should not obstruct the driver's view of the road scene nor should it obstruct vehicle controls and displays required for the primary driving task. It should be designed such that allocation of driver attention to the system displays and controls remains compatible with the demand of the driving situation.

- Issues related to privacy of the data acquired by the device (i.e., who has access to data) must be considered.

- Acceptance or "buy-in" from stakeholders—drivers, fleet operators/managers, trucking associations, and labor unions—must be obtained.

- Issues related to automatic vs. manual activation and deactivation of the device must be considered.

3. SUMMARY AND ASSESSMENT OF FATIGUE DETECTION AND MONITORING TECHNOLOGIES

Technological approaches have continued to emerge in recent years that hold promise for detecting and monitoring dangerous levels of driver drowsiness. While some enduring systems and devices have been available as prototypes for a decade or more, many of these technologies are now in the development, validation testing, or early implementation stages. Previous studies have reviewed available fatigue detection and prediction technologies and methodologies (Krueger 2004; Hartley et al. 2000). This paper builds on previous work by providing updated information on state-of-the-art emerging fatigue detection and alertness monitoring technologies. Significant advances in video camera and computer processing technologies coupled with robust, non-invasive eye detection and tracking systems have made it possible to characterize and monitor a driver's state of alertness in real time under all types of driving conditions. In this section, some currently available drowsy driver monitoring devices, as well as technologies that will be available in the near future for commercial transport applications, are identified and described. This information was compiled using a combination of several methods, including literature searches of technical and scientific journals as well as the Internet, e-mail, and phone correspondence with researchers, engineers, and product managers involved in developing these technologies, and on-site visits and technical demonstrations. In each case, the information presented is categorized in terms of the device's background, functionality, and use; relevant research findings; and future directions for device development. It is also noted if no information was available to fit a particular heading.

3.1   ATTENTION TECHNOLOGY, INC.

3.1.1   Device Background, Functionality, and Use

Attention Technology, Inc. has designed and developed the DD850 Driver Fatigue Monitor (DFM), the only real-time, on-board drowsiness monitor that is currently being tested in an extensive field operational test. The DFM is a video-based drowsiness detection system for measuring slow eyelid closure. It is designed to mount on the vehicle's dashboard just to the right of the steering wheel, and it provides a continuous real-time measurement of eye position and eyelid closure (Grace 2001; Bierman et al. 1999). The camera module is mounted on a rotating base to allow the driver to adjust the camera angle. The field of view is large enough to accommodate normal head movement. The device has a visual gauge that represents the driver's drowsiness level and emits an audible warning when the driver reaches a preset drowsiness threshold. The gauge employs six light-emitting diodes (LEDs); the first three LEDs are amber, representing moderate drowsiness levels, and the second three are red, representing severe drowsiness. With a three-stage alarm, the device provides real-time, immediate feedback to the driver. The DFM is pictured in Figure 1.

Specifically, the DFM estimates PERCLOS, which is the proportion of time the eyes are closed 80% or more over a specified time interval. PERCLOS has been demonstrated in both driving and non-driving tasks to be a valid indicator of drowsiness and performance degradation due to drowsiness.

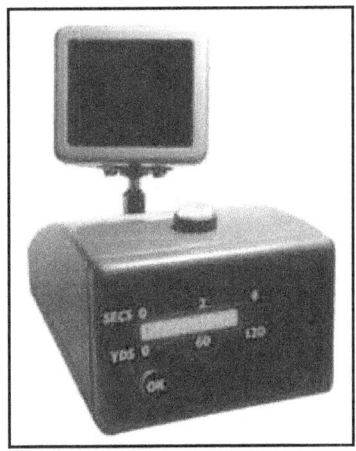

**Figure 1. Attention Technology DD850
Driver Fatigue Monitor**

The DFM uses a structured illumination approach to identify the driver's eyes (Grace). This approach obtains two coUcutive images of the driver using a single camera. The first image is acquired using an infrared (IR) illumination source that produces a bright-eye image (i.e., a distinct glowing) of the driver's pupils. The second image uses an IR illumination source at different wavelength to produce an image with dark pupils. These two images are essentially identical except for the brightness of the pupils in the image. A third image calculates the difference of these two images, enhancing the bright eyes and eliminating all image features except for the bright pupils. The driver's eyes are identified in this third image by applying a threshold to the pixel brightness. The bright pupil effect utilized by the DFM is a simple and effective eye tracking approach for pupil detection based on a differential lighting scheme. The high contrast between the pupils and the rest of the face can significantly improve the eye tracking robustness and accuracy. However, this technique also has disadvantages and limitations.

3.1.2   Research Findings

The success of the bright pupil technique strongly depends on the brightness and size of the pupils, which are often functions of face orientation, external illumination interference, and the distance of the subject from the camera (Liu et al. 2002). For real-world, in-vehicle applications, sunlight can interfere with IR illumination, reflections from eyeglasses can create confounding bright spots near the eyes, and sunglasses tend to disturb the IR light and make the pupils appear very weak. Thus, the DFM is intended for use in commercial operations involving nighttime driving.

An on-road FOT of the DFM, co-sponsored by FMCSA and the National Highway Traffic Safety Administration (NHTSA), is currently in progress to determine the safety benefits of using the device to measure the alertness of commercial truck drivers. The FOT consists of 37 vehicles equipped with the device and 102 truck drivers, each driving for 17 weeks.

3.1.3   Future Directions

None specified.

3.2   DELPHI ELECTRONICS AND SAFETY

3.2.1   Device Background, Functionality, and Use

Delphi is currently developing an automotive-grade, real-time, vision-based driver state monitoring system that aims to improve safety by preventing drivers from falling asleep or from being overly distracted. According to a corporate white paper (GJ Witt, personal communication, 2005), the system integrates two products, the ForeWarn Drowsy Driver Alert and the ForeWarn Driver Distraction Alert, into a comprehensive Driver State Monitor (DSM). The DSM is a computer vision system that uses a single camera mounted on the dashboard directly in front of the driver and two IR illumination sources. The installation is shown in Figure 2. This figure shows the camera mounted on top of the dashboard directly above the center of the steering wheel and one of the IR illumination sources embedded in the dashboard next to the speedometer on the right side of the steering wheel. Upon detecting and tracking the driver's facial features, the system analyzes eye closures and head pose to infer fatigue or distraction level. While Delphi considered drowsiness and distraction measures other than the ones based on computer vision (driving performance and heart/respiration rates, for example), computer vision was regarded as the preferred approach because it offers the most direct indication of early oUt of sleepiness and distraction, and is also seen as an excellent platform to be shared with other vision-based driver assistance applications in the future.

The DSM evaluates eye closures and the forward attention level of the driver over time using a single high-fidelity imaging sensor. The camera and the near-IR illumination sources are unobtrusive, and the system provides feedback regarding the driver's distraction and drowsiness levels as well as an audible warning alert. It provides extended eye-closure warning for closures longer than 2.5 seconds, and it also provides extended distraction warning for non-forward gaze states in excess of 2.5 seconds. The system also features automatic driver detection (self-calibration) and does not require training. The oUt of fatigue is detected before the driver falls asleep at the wheel.

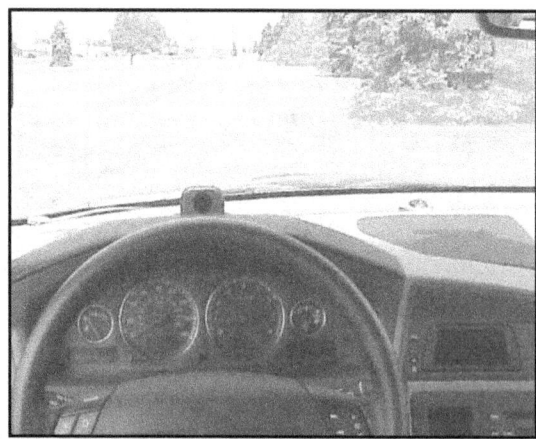

Figure 2. Delphi DSM Installed in Vehicle

The fatigue detection algorithm predicts AVECLOS, the percentage of time the eyes are estimated to be fully closed over a one-minute interval. AVECLOS is a simple binary measure indicating whether or not the driver's eyes are fully closed. This is a less complex measure of drowsiness than PERCLOS, and, as a result, it permits the use of an automotive-grade data processor as opposed to a high-grade PC processor required for PERCLOS. Validation testing at Delphi has shown very close correlation between AVECLOS and PERCLOS (Pearson correlation coefficient = 0.95).

3.2.2   Research Findings

DSM is being developed for the automobile and commercial vehicle market; thus it is critical to ensure that the system works in a real-world automotive environment. Some of the automotive requirements addressed during the design and development of DSM included a wide range of illumination conditions and operating temperatures, coverage of the 95th percentile ellipsoid of driver head positions, available camera locations, system cost, heat dissipation, allowable levels of IR irradiation, and subject variability. The production version of DSM will not have a display, though the configuration currently being used for experimental testing and product development incorporates a display showing a video image of the driver's face/head and eye tracking region as well as color-coded outputs regarding levels of distraction and fatigue. The display is pictured in Figure 3, showing the driver's face with his eyes closed and the red bars on the feedback monitor indicating a severe level of fatigue. The DSM is presently installed in a Volvo demonstration vehicle, where it has been shown to be a reliable predictor of drowsiness under all illumination conditions and for drivers wearing eyeglasses and most types of sunglasses.

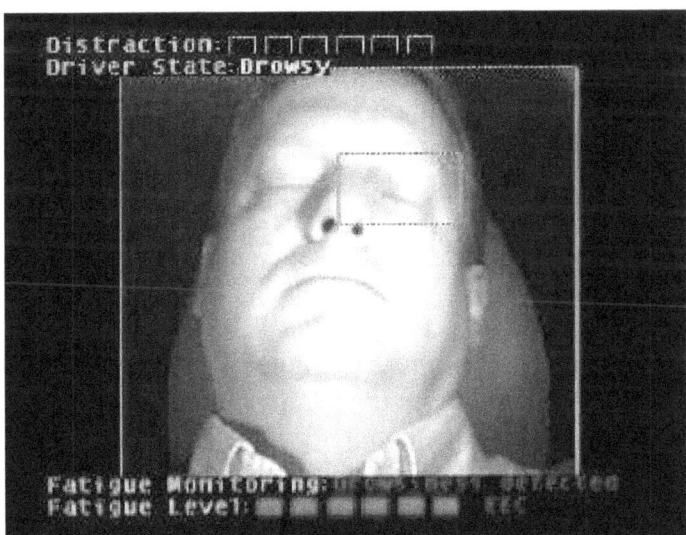

Figure 3. Delphi DSM In-Vehicle Display

3.2.3   Future Directions

None specified.

3.3   SEEING MACHINES

3.3.1   Device Background, Functionality, and Use

Seeing Machines is engaged in the research, development, and production of advanced computer vision systems for research in human performance measurement, advanced driver assistance systems, transportation, biometric acquisition, situational awareness, robotics, and medical applications. As described in product information on their website (www.seeingmachines.com/facelab.htm), their signature product, faceLAB™, provides head and face tracking as well as eye, eyelid, and gaze tracking for human subjects using a non-contact, video-based sensor. faceLAB™ has a flexible and mobile tracking system and a wide field of view that enables analysis of naturalistic behavior, including head pose, gaze direction, and eyelid closure, in real time under real-world conditions without the use of wires, magnets, or headgear. Thus, it is a tool that has great promise for analyzing driver behavior in simulators and test vehicles.

Drowsiness can be determined in real time with faceLAB's comprehensive blink analysis and PERCLOS assessment, including delivery of raw data on the details of eyelid behavior. Measurements are taken on eyelid position, rather than bright pupil or corneal occlusion. Instead of using traditional corneal reflection techniques, input is obtained using a stereo camera pair. In addition, faceLAB™ allows each subject to be automatically calibrated, and the data are reusable in subsequent experiments.

Seeing Machines' faceLAB™ has been employed extensively as a PC-based research tool. It is installed in several driving simulators, including the National Advanced Driving Simulator at the University of Iowa and at the University of Minnesota, and it has been used in test track experiments at NHTSA's Vehicle Research Test Center. In addition, a single-camera system is installed on a Volvo Safety Truck demonstration vehicle. The PC-based version of faceLAB™ is shown in Figure 4, which depicts a person facing a computer monitor that displays his face and a close-up view of his eyes along with six graphs showing the real-time device output. The two cameras are attached to a mounting bracket just below the computer monitor and are aimed directly at the person's face. The two-camera system installed in a vehicle for road testing is shown in Figure 5. The two cameras and the IR illuminator are clearly visible mounted on the dashboard above the steering wheel.

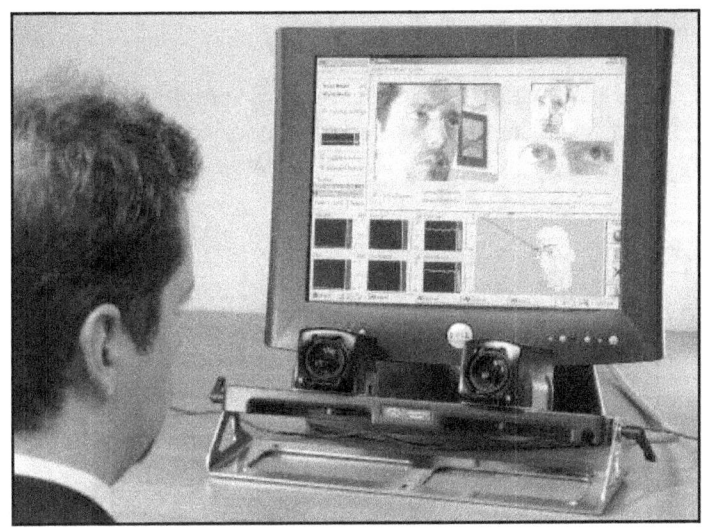

Figure 4. Seeing Machines faceLAB™

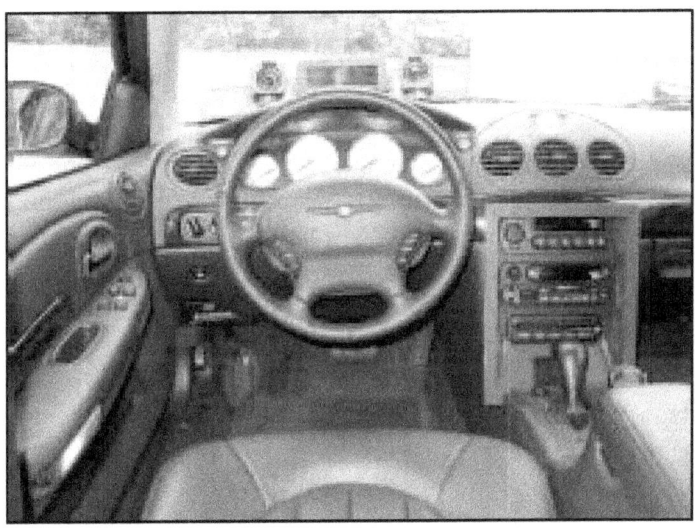

Figure 5. faceLAB™ Installation in Vehicle

3.3.2   Research Findings

faceLAB™ operates and maintains tracking integrity through a range of lighting and movement conditions. It is not sensitive to sudden movement or obstruction, and it recovers immediately if a subject leaves the field of view. The device reportedly works in bright sunlight or at night, with subjects close to the camera or several feet away. It also works with or without contact leUs and with most eyeglasses. For example, if the subject is wearing sunglasses and his eyes cannot be seen, faceLAB™ can still find the head pose, eyes, and mouth, and can, according to Seeing Machines, continue to produce reliable data. The device reportedly works very well in the simulator environment.

3.3.3 Future Directions

Currently, Seeing Machines is developing a prototype in-vehicle system for Volkswagen that will include a warning alert feature and will be tested under real-world conditions. The prototype will be available in approximately one year.

3.4 SMART EYE AB

3.4.1 Device Background, Functionality, and Use

Smart Eye AB, headquartered in Göteborg, Sweden, was formed in 1999 with a mission to provide the general public, industry, and research institutions with computer-vision-based software that enables computers and machines to detect human face/head movement, eye movement, and gaze direction. Online product information in 2006 (www.smarteye.se/downloads.aspx) indicated that Smart Eye has developed and tested Smart Eye Pro 3.0, a remote and unobtrusive sensor that measures face and eye movement for a variety of applications, including transportation safety research (drowsiness, alertness) and simulators.

Smart Eye Pro 3.0 is a machine vision system that estimates head pose using a simple and robust method based on tracking of individual facial features and a three-dimensional (3D) head model. The initial head model is generic and adapted to the user. The head modeling is initialized using a simple step-by-step application in which the user benchmarks basic and prominent features (e.g., nose, mouth) in the face images. Once the system runs in tracking mode, the 3D feature locations are determined from their previous locations and a motion model. If tracking is suddenly lost, a fast face detection procedure allows the system to quickly re-acquire the subject's face and resume tracking. While the face is being tracked, gaze direction and eyelid positions are determined by combining image edge information with 3D models of the eye and eyelids. The system is flexible and can accommodate up to four high-speed 60-Hz cameras. Thus, a major advantage is that eye and head tracking can continue even if one camera is fully occluded or otherwise non-operational. This also allows for large head motions (translation and rotation). Another important property of the system is that it is easily adaptable to various measurement situations with flexible camera mount positions. Smart Eye manufactures the image-processing based sensor but does not develop an algorithm that monitors drowsiness. To support a validation test, Smart Eye could provide a PERCLOS algorithm along with their camera system.

3.4.2 Research Findings

Smart Eye Pro 3.0 is able to provide accurate eye tracking under all illumination conditions, from bright sunlight to complete darkness, by using an innovative active IR lighting approach that suppresses the effects of sunlight and shadows. It also reportedly works well for drivers who have low-contrast eyes and who wear contact leUs, eyeglasses, and most types of sunglasses.

A system consisting of a single camera and PC-based processor is currently being tested in Europe by Volvo, Volkswagen, BMW, and all the European truck manufacturers. Smart Eye reports that they have been receiving very favorable reviews from these on-road field tests with regard to the system's ability to monitor the driver's eye and head movement and gaze direction in both sunlight and darkness, as well as for drivers wearing eyeglasses.

3.4.3   Future Directions

Smart Eye's long-term plan is to go into serial production and have the device available as an option for the automobile market in three years.

3.5   SENSOMOTORIC INSTRUMENTS GMBH

3.5.1   Device Background, Functionality, and Use

SensoMotoric Instruments GmbH (SMI), based in Berlin, Germany, is currently developing InSight™, an advanced, non-invasive, computer-vision-based operator monitoring system that measures head position and orientation, gaze direction, eyelid opening, and pupil position and diameter. Product information provided to the authors via e-mail (E. Schmidt, personal communication, 2005) shows that it is a high-speed system that uses a sampling rate of 120 Hz for head pose and gaze measurement, 120 Hz for eyelid closure and blink measurement, and 60 Hz for combined gaze, head pose, and eyelid measurement. To determine a driver's state of alertness, InSight™ calculates PERCLOS. The system is purported to employ automatic and robust tracking algorithms that allow accurate driver state monitoring under all lighting conditions from sunlight to darkness. The system also features very simple and fast user calibration to accommodate multiple drivers.

Figure 6 shows the InSight™ system setup for in-vehicle driver monitoring. The photo is taken from the passenger side of the vehicle and shows the driver seated with his hands on the steering wheel and the camera and IR illumination hardware mounted on the dashboard above the steering wheel. The present configuration is a PC-based system that uses one high-speed, dashboard-mounted camera and three sources of low-intensity controlled IR illumination. The system provides a comparatively large tracking range because it uses a small tracking area on the face (eye and nose features only) for measuring head/face position and orientation. Their system is suitable for 24-hour operation. It measures head position and orientation, eye position, and eyelid closure for a more refined prediction of PERCLOS, and subsequently driver drowsiness.

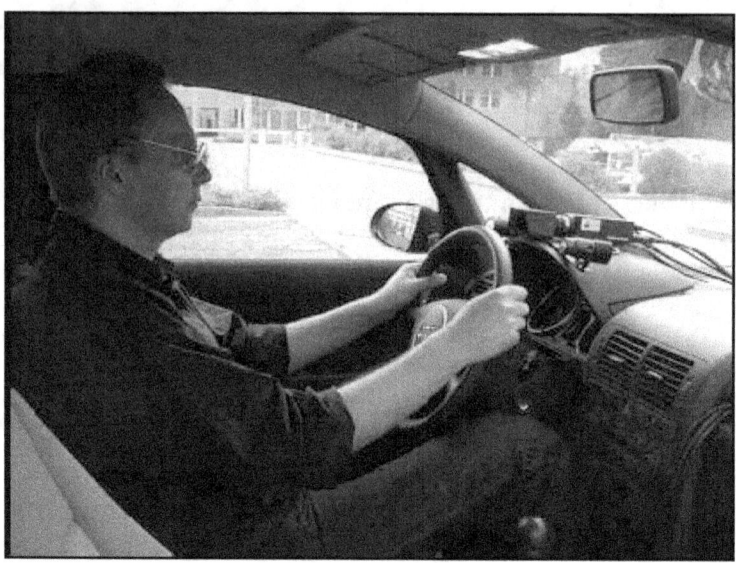

Figure 6. SMI InSight™ Driver Monitoring System Setup

3.5.2   Research Findings

The eye closure measurement accuracy is 1 mm. As mentioned, InSight™ is currently a PC-based research platform, although extensive studies have been conducted with truck drivers and passenger cars. SMI has also conducted studies comparing simulator and on-road performance to detect drowsiness and micro-sleeps. They have been working with Volkswagen and BMW to test the device in the real-world driving environment.

3.5.3   Future Directions

SMI's plan was to partner with an OEM by the summer of 2005 to develop the technology into a production-quality, automotive-based drowsiness detection and monitoring system.

3.6   APPLIED SCIENCE LABORATORIES

3.6.1   Device Background, Functionality, and Use

Applied Science Laboratories (ASL) has been designing and developing eye tracking systems and devices for over 30 years for applications in fields such as human factors and ergonomics, marketing research, psychology and cognition, and education and training. According to product information provided to the authors (V. Salem, personal communication, 2005) their video-based eye trackers utilize the pupil/corneal reflection technique for measuring eye movements. In most applications, ASL devices operate with a bright pupil image. This has been chosen because of the advantages it provides over a dark pupil image. ASL has found that the bright pupil image is less affected by eyelashes, light-colored eyes, dark environments, contact leUs, eyeglasses, and distance from the camera. On the other hand, a disadvantage of the bright-pupil technique is that it is not as robust in an outdoor environment, since sunlight can interfere with infrared illumination. In those cases, ASL uses a specially enhanced dark-pupil technique in which the optics are designed specifically for outdoor use and are robust even in bright sunlight.

Many of ASL's eye tracking devices for outdoor applications (including in-vehicle driving purposes) utilize a camera mounted on an adjustable, lightweight headband. These devices provide unrestricted freedom of movement and can accommodate all types of subjects including those wearing sunglasses, but nevertheless may be considered rather obtrusive. ASL does, however, manufacture a remote, non-contacting eye tracking system better suited for in-vehicle, real-time monitoring of driver alertness. This system, the ETS-PC II, is pictured in Figure 7, which shows the eye tracker secured to the dashboard above the center console to the right of the steering wheel.

The ASL technology that is developed for in-vehicle transportation applications is primarily a PC-based research instrument. The camera-based system is non-invasive, but the computer must be present in the vehicle to process the data. Also, the eye tracking system does not include an algorithm for detecting and alerting a drowsy driver.

3.6.2   Research Findings

The ETS-PC II, is designed to provide a full 90° horizontal and 45° vertical field of view for accurate measurement of the driver's eye movement and line of sight. The eye is reliably reacquired if the head is turned over 90° and then returns. It features automatic and continuous search for the eye as well as automatic head movement compensation and parallax correction. Furthermore, the system can reportedly integrate eye gaze data with a time stamp to other data signals from the vehicle, such as steering position or vehicle speed. ASL states that the device works in all driving conditions from bright sunlight to total darkness.

3.6.3   Future Directions

None specified.

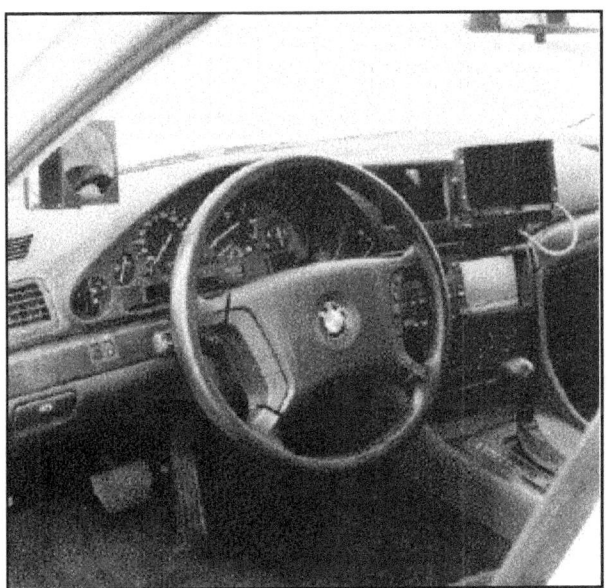

Figure 7. ASL ETS-PC II In-Vehicle Eye Tracking System

3.7 LC TECHNOLOGIES, INC.

3.7.1 Device Background, Functionality, and Use

LC Technologies, Inc. has developed an eye tracking technology that is both an eye-operated computer for control and communication and a device for monitoring and recording eye motion and related eye data (Cleveland 1999). Product information available online (www.eyegaze.com) in 2006 indicate that the technology, called the Eyegaze Analysis System, is a hands-off, unobtrusive, remote human-computer interface that can be used to track a user's gaze point or allow an operator to interact with his or her environment using only his or her eyes. The device reportedly has a number of human factors research applications, including monitoring mental alertness and determining fitness for duty.

The Eyegaze Analysis System is a tool for measuring, recording, playing back, and analyzing what a person is doing with his/her eyes. It includes all the basic video equipment, computer hardware, and Eyegaze software necessary to develop and run custom eye tracking applications. In the laboratory, gaze point tracking measurements are made unobtrusively via a remote video camera mounted below a computer monitor. The Eyegaze Analysis System tracks the subject's gaze point on the screen automatically and in real time, with gaze point measurements made at a rate of 60 Hz. Gaze direction is determined using the Pupil Center Corneal Reflection (PCCR) method. A small, low-power infrared LED located at the center of the camera lens illuminates the eye and provides a direct reflection off the cornea of the eye.

For its use as a drowsy driver detection and warning system, the Eyegaze Analysis System can be housed in the vehicle cab to warn and alert drivers when they are becoming drowsy and losing alertness on the road. The goal of the system is to monitor the driver's eye point-of-regard, saccadic and fixation activity, and percentage eyelid closure reliably, in real time, and under all anticipated driving conditions. Recent effort at LC Technologies has been directed toward developing the camera/sensor instrument, but no significant work has been done to advance the Eyegaze Analysis System for transportation applications.

3.7.2 Research Findings

The concept for the Driver Eye Monitor is for the miniature video camera to be mounted on a motorized gimbal that keeps the camera pointed at and focused on the eye. The camera must have a clear, unobstructed view of the subject's eye to make an accurate gaze measurement. In most cases, eye tracking works with eyeglasses and contact leUs since the calibration procedure accounts for the refractive properties of the leUs. However, eyeglasses tilted significantly downward, hard contact leUs, and sunglasses may cause problems for the device by reflecting the LED off the surface of the glass back into the camera. In addition, sunlight contains high levels of infrared light and obscures the lighting from the device's LED, degrading the image of the eye.

It has been tested in a real-world environment on LC Technologies' RV platform; however, the purpose of the test was to track the eye movements of the passenger, who was attempting to operate a computer with the eyes only in a hands-free mode. The device has not been validated against any measures of driver drowsiness such as PERCLOS or eye gaze behavior. It reportedly works well in sunlight and for drivers who wear most types of sunglasses (reflective sunglasses present a problem).

3.7.3 Future Directions

None specified.

3.8 JOHNS HOPKINS UNIVERSITY APPLIED PHYSICS LABORATORY

3.8.1 Device Background, Functionality, and Use

Johns Hopkins University Applied Physics Laboratory (2005) is developing a small sensor system that will alert drivers when they are in danger of falling asleep at the wheel or experiencing some level of impairment from fatigue. The Drowsy Driver Detection System (DDDS) is a device containing a transceiver similar to those used in automatic door entry systems that operate at safe microwave frequency and power levels. It detects drowsiness prior to the driver's falling asleep. It issues warnings that can begin as the driver becomes sleepy and intensify as the system detects increasing drowsiness. The system is non-invasive and it collects specific driver data under all conditions, including bright sunlight, through the use of a Doppler radar system. The technique can monitor and quantitatively measure the speed, frequency, and duration of eyelid closure, rate of heartbeat and respiration, and pulse rate by analyzing the Doppler components in the reflected signal.

The final design size of the DDDS is projected to be approximately $3\times3\times2$ inches for the transceiver (small enough to fit above the windshield) and about $1\times2\times3$ inches for the support electronics. Based on the relatively simple design of the system and the projected low cost of production, the device is expected to be cost-effective to use. This technology is appealing from the standpoint of its ability to unobtrusively monitor driver behavior under all types of driving conditions and for all drivers. However, the technology has not advanced beyond the basic research phase of development.

3.8.2 Research Findings

Testing has shown good correlation between measurements obtained with the DDDS and those taken using the validated PERCLOS methodology. But it should be noted that these tests were performed on only one subject.

3.8.3 Future Directions

Substantial additional work to develop the algorithm, collect data in the laboratory on several experimental subjects, and correlate the device output to a validated measure of drowsiness such as PERCLOS is required before a prototype system will be ready for real-world testing.

3.9   RENSSELAER POLYTECHNIC INSTITUTE

3.9.1   Device Background, Functionality, and Use

Researchers at Rensselaer Polytechnic Institute (RPI) have developed a prototype computer vision system for monitoring driver vigilance (Ji et al. 2004; Ji et al. 2005; Ji and Yang 2002). The main components of the system include a remotely located charge coupled device (CCD) video camera, a specially designed hardware system for real-time image acquisition and for controlling the illuminator and alarm system, and various computer vision algorithms for simultaneous, real-time non-intrusive monitoring of various visual bio-behaviors that typically characterize a driver's level of vigilance.

Many current approaches and systems that use computer vision technologies for extracting characteristics of a driver focus on using only a single visual cue such as eyelid movement, line of sight, or head orientation to characterize the driver's state of alertness. The system relying on a single visual cue may encounter difficulty when the required visual features cannot be acquired accurately or reliably. For example, eyeglasses can cause glare and may be opaque to light, making it impossible for a camera to monitor eye movement. Another potential problem with the use of a single visual cue is that the obtained visual feature may not always be indicative of a driver's state of mental alertness. For example, an irregular head movement or gaze direction (e.g., briefly looking behind or at the rear-view mirror) may potentially produce a false alarm for such a system. RPI contends that all those visual cues, however imperfect they may be individually, if combined systematically can reduce the uncertainty and ambiguity in the information from a single source and provide an accurate characterization of a driver's level of vigilance. Thus, the system they are developing can simultaneously and unobtrusively monitor in real time several visual behaviors that typically characterize a person's level of alertness while driving. These visual cues include eyelid and gaze movement, pupil movement, head movement, and facial expression. The parameters computed from these visual cues are subsequently combined probabilistically using a Bayesian Networks model to form a composite index that can robustly, accurately, and consistently characterize a driver's alertness level.

Eye detection and tracking are accomplished using active near-infrared illumination to brighten the subject's face to produce the bright pupil effect. This ensures a high-quality image under varying real-world conditions, including poor illumination, daylight, and darkness, and it minimizes any interference with the subject's ability to drive. For implementation of their system in a vehicle, RPI proposes to use two miniature CCD cameras embedded on the dashboard. The first camera is a narrow-angle camera focused on the driver's eyes to monitor eyelid and gaze movements, and the second camera is a wide-angle camera aimed at the driver's head to track and monitor head movement and facial expression. There are several ocular measures to characterize eyelid movement, such as eye blink frequency, eye closure duration, eye closure speed, and PERCLOS.

The RPI computer vision system focuses on real-time computation of PERCLOS and average eye closure speed (AECS) to characterize eye movement. While PERCLOS is purported to be the most valid ocular parameter for measuring driver drowsiness, studies at RPI indicate that AECS differs for drowsy versus alert subjects and is therefore also a potentially useful and valid indicator of driver drowsiness. In addition to measuring eyelid movement, RPI has developed

24

methods for determining three-dimensional face (head) orientation, eye gaze estimation and tracking, and facial expression (e.g., mouth movement, yawning). All these measures are potentially valuable in detecting a driver's level of alertness and attention. The prototype of RPI's fatigue monitor, showing the images from the eye and face cameras, as well as the real-time output of the composite fatigue index, is presented in Figure 8.

3.9.2   Research Findings

Experimental studies in a simulated (laboratory) environment under various illumination conditions—using eight subjects (both in a rested, alert condition and in a sleep-deprived condition) of different genders, ages, and ethnic backgrounds—were conducted to validate the drowsiness monitoring system. The validation consisted of two parts; the first involved the validation of the measurement accuracy of their computer vision techniques, and the second assessed the validity of the parameters that were computed to characterize drowsiness. Subjects were asked to perform a Test of Variables Attention (TOVA), a 20-minute psychomotor reaction test requiring the subjects to sustain attention and respond to a randomly appearing light on a computer screen by pressing a button. From the validation tests, RPI researchers found that: (1) PERCLOS and TOVA respoU time were closely correlated; (2) their fatigue monitor accurately measured PERCLOS, a valid characterization and predictor of drowsiness; and (3) the composite fatigue index computed by their fatigue algorithm was highly correlated with the subject's TOVA respoU time. On the basis of these experimental results, it was concluded that this monitor system is reasonably robust, reliable, and accurate in characterizing and predicting human drowsiness.

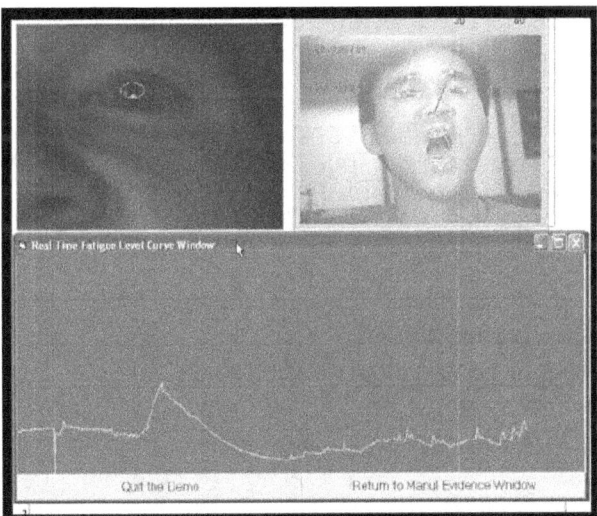

Figure 8. RPI Fatigue Monitor Prototype

3.9.3   Future Directions

RPI has conducted both basic research and algorithm development. Their technological approach and prototype are promising, but limited to the laboratory environment. To advance their technology to a workable, on-board, automotive-grade system, RPI would need to collaborate with an industry partner.

25

3.10   THE GEORGE WASHINGTON UNIVERSITY

3.10.1   Device Background, Functionality, and Use

Researchers at The George Washington University's (GWU) Center for Intelligent System Research are developing a method for detecting drowsiness in drivers based on an Artificial Neural Network (ANN) (Sayed et al. 2001; Eskandarian and Sayed 2005). The ANN observes the steering angle patterns and classifies them into drowsy- and non-drowsy-driving intervals. Unlike other drowsiness detection systems that are based on measuring driver physical and/or physiological data (EEG data and eye movements, for example) and that require obtrusive wires, cameras, monitors, or other devices attached to or aimed at the driver, the ANN method measures and analyzes vehicle performance output data only. Thus, because of the non-invasive nature of this method and because it is not dependent on environmental conditions such as ambient light, neural network technology is potentially a very practical method for in-vehicle 24-hour fatigue/drowsiness monitoring.

Neural networks are very sophisticated nonlinear modeling techniques capable of modeling extremely complex functions. Neural networks are relatively easy to use compared with other types of nonlinear statistical models. With their ability to derive meaning from complicated or imprecise data, they can be used to extract patterns and detect trends that are too complex to be noticed either by humans or by other computer techniques.

Steering wheel movements have been of particular interest in studies of driver alertness. Various researchers have shown that changes in steering activity, computed over fixed time intervals, are correlated with a driver's state of impairment. The hypothesized relationship between driver state of alertness and steering wheel position is that, in an alert state, drivers make small amplitude movements of the steering wheel, corresponding to small adjustments in vehicle trajectory; in a drowsy state, on the other hand, these steering wheel movements become less precise and larger in amplitude, resulting in sharp changes in trajectory.

3.10.2   Research Findings

GWU researchers trained and tested the ANN by conducting a driving simulator experiment. Twelve drivers, each under a different level of sleep deprivation, were tested. Results showed that the ANN method detected drowsiness with an accuracy of 90%. On several occasions during the simulator experiment, drivers fell asleep while driving and crashed the vehicle. For all the crashes that occurred, a data set representing 3.5 minutes of driving immediately preceding the crash was presented to the ANN. The ANN detected drowsy-driving behavior before the crash occurred and generated a warning in all cases.

3.10.3   Future Directions

This technology is still in the early research stage of development. Based on the work completed thus far, researchers at GWU have identified and recommended the following areas for further research:

- Conduct further refining and validation of the algorithm

- Capture an individual driver's steering activity while drowsy

- Conduct additional simulator experiments to validate the algorithm, test additional road conditions, and test a more diversified group of drivers

- Test the ANN technology on the road in an instrumented vehicle, and refine the algorithm based on the road test data

- Conduct research on warning systems integrated with the detection system

3.11   FORD MOTOR COMPANY

Ford Motor Company is currently teaming with Volvo to develop an in-vehicle unobtrusive fatigue monitoring system. The system is being developed for use in passenger vehicles, but could be adapted to the commercial vehicle platform. Ford is currently in the patent application process and could not, therefore, disclose any details of the system's technology approach or operating principles. They did state, however, that their device would be ready for on-road testing in about one year.

The framework presented in the two tables below provides a straightforward means of comparing and contrasting the various technologies described in this paper. As an example, the technologies, presented in the table columns, are evaluated against a number of criteria listed in the rows—the major scientific/engineering guidelines, in Table 2, and the major user acceptance elements in Table 3. The single, capital letters in the grids indicate whether the device meets the criterion: a **Y** means "Yes," the device meets the criterion; an **N** means "No," the device does not meet the criterion; and a **U** is for "Undetermined," meaning that that the criterion has not been scientifically evaluated and more data are needed.

Table 2. Technology Comparison and Criteria Evaluation—Scientific Engineering Guidelines
(Key—to whether criterion has been met: Y=Yes, N=No, U=Undetermined)

Scientific/ Engineering Guidelines	Criteria	Attention Technology Driver Fatigue Monitor	Delphi Driver State Monitor	Seeing Machines faceLAB™	Smart Eye Pro 3.0	SMI InSight™	ASL ETS-PC II	LC Tech. Eyegaze Analysis System	Johns Hopkins APL DDDS	RPI Prototype Fatigue Monitor	GWU Artificial Neural Network
Environmental	Device should operate reliably and accurately in all illumination conditions	N	U	U	U	U	U	U	U	U	Y
Environmental	Device should operate over expected range of truck cab temperature, humidity, and vibration conditions	Y	Y	Y	Y	Y	Y	Y	U	U	U
Reliability	Device should be designed to minimize both missed events and false alarms	U	U	U	U	U	U	U	U	U	U
Anthropometric	Device should accommodate multiple drivers with minimal re-calibration	Y	Y	Y	Y	Y	U	U	U	Y	Y
Engineering Design	Device should be robust and require only normal maintenance and replacement	U	U	U	U	U	U	U	U	U	U

28

Table 3. Technology Comparison and Criteria Evaluation—User Acceptance Elements

(Key—to whether criterion has been met: Y=Yes, N=No, U=Undetermined)

User Acceptance Elements	Criteria	Attention Technology Driver Fatigue Monitor	Delphi Driver State Monitor	Seeing Machines faceLAB™	Smart Eye Pro 3.0	SMI InSight™	ASL ETS-PC II	LC Tech. Eyegaze Analysis System	Johns Hopkins APL DDDS	RPI Prototype Fatigue Monitor	GWU Artificial Neural Network
Ease of Use	Device must not be invasive	Y	Y	Y	Y	Y	Y	Y	Y	Y	Y
Ease of Use	Device must accommodate corrective eyeglasses and most types of sunglasses	N	Y	Y	Y	Y	U	U	U	U	Y
Ease of Use	Device should present a warning alert to the driver	Y	Y	Y	Y	Y	N	N	N	Y	N
Ease of Use	Device must monitor driver behavior in real time	Y	Y	Y	Y	Y	Y	Y	Y	Y	Y
Ease of Use	Device should require minimal training	Y	Y	Y	Y	Y	Y	Y	Y	Y	Y
Ease of Learning	Assessment of the time it takes users to feel proficient with the device	U	U	U	U	U	U	U	U	U	U
Ease of Learning	Assessment of user ability to retain and recall information regarding device functionality	U	U	U	U	U	U	U	U	U	U
Perceived Value	Device should provide feedback to driver regarding alertness level	Y	Y	U	U	U	N	N	U	Y	U

User Acceptance Elements	Criteria	Attention Technology Driver Fatigue Monitor	Delphi Driver State Monitor	Seeing Machines faceLAB™	Smart Eye Pro 3.0	SMI InSight™	ASL ETS-PC II	LC Tech. Eyegaze Analysis System	Johns Hopkins APL DDDS	RPI Prototype Fatigue Monitor	GWU Artificial Neural Network
Perceived Value	Is there a perceived safety benefit or increased risk associated with device use?	U	U	U	U	U	U	U	U	U	U
Advocacy	Assessment of user's intent to purchase device	U	U	U	U	U	U	U	U	U	U
Advocacy	Willingness of user to recommend device use to others	U	U	U	U	U	U	U	U	U	U
Driver Behavior	Device must not distract the driver from driving task or from responding to other safety devices	Y	Y	Y	Y	Y	Y	Y	Y	Y	Y
Driver Behavior	Assessment of behavioral adaptation to the device over time	U	U	U	U	U	U	U	U	U	U

30

4. UPDATE ON EMERGING TECHNOLOGIES: ADVANCED SENSOR DEVELOPMENT FOR ATTENTION, STRESS, VIGILANCE, AND SLEEP/WAKEFULNESS MONITORING

The Advanced Sensor Development for Attention, Stress, Vigilance and Sleep/Wakefulness Monitoring (SENSATION) project is a four-year, 17-million-Euro effort focused on exploring a wide range of micro and nanosensor technologies, with the aim of achieving unobtrusive, cost-effective, real-time monitoring, detection, and prediction of human physiological state in relation to wakefulness, fatigue, and stress anytime, everywhere, and for everybody (Bekiaris et al. 2004b). The SENSATION Consortium consists of 45 partners in academia and industry from 20 countries in the European Union (EU), Australia, and China covering the following research areas: brain-sensing, neurosensing, computational neuroscience, signal processing, materials science, optoelectronics, microelectronics, intelligent user interfaces, telematics, data fusion, sleep research, human physiological measurements, and clinical/medical research.

The stated specific goals of the SENSATION project are to design, develop, and extensively test two new nanosensors and 17 new miniaturized microsensors to monitor, predict, and detect human physiological states (Bekiaris et al. 2004b). A decision was made to apply this project to the issue of sleepy drivers. Transportation-related project objectives include the following:

- Definition of sleep/wakefulness and their transition states, as well as stress, inattention, and emotional states, by a set of measurable criteria and their correlation with measurement methodologies and tools

- Modeling of sleep stages and extraction of requirements and specifications for sensors to measure the required model parameters

- Development of nano and microsensor technologies for unobtrusive monitoring of physiological state and activity

- Development of camera-based microsensors for high-precision, cost-efficient, and high-speed measurement of EOG and motility parameters and estimation of the person's vigilance and attention state

- Development of posture and capacitive microsensors for measurement of physiological and activity-related parameters to estimate the person's vigilance and attention state

- Development of eyelid and skin micro and nanosensors for respiration and skin conductivity measurements (autonomic functions) to estimate the person's sleep/wakefulness state and analyze its characteristics (i.e., differentiating normal from abnormal sleep)

- Development of innovative signal processing and computational intelligence algorithms for data fusion, data management, sensor integration, and power consumption minimization

- Development of user-friendly, modular, and intuitive user interfaces for sensor output presentation as well as for real-time warnings to the user in case a problem is detected

- Development of a multi-purpose sensing platform to assess the physiological state of a user that will be: autonomous (will operate in real time, continuously monitoring the user); non-supervised (diagnosis will be displayed to the user without any on-line intervention from an expert); non-intrusive (no wires or cables so that the subject is not overly aware of the system); and robust (will function in an unpredictable real-world environment where conditions cannot be controlled)

To summarize, the SENSATION project uses a multisensor platform approach to the problem of sleepiness and fatigue-related workplace accidents, with an intended outcome of improved worker health, safety, and quality of life. This will be accomplished through the novel use of micro and nanosensors and related technologies, at low cost and high efficiency, for physiological state monitoring (Bekiaris et al. 2004b). As this report was being written, the EU planned to start a research program in 2007 to foster innovation and competitiveness. This European technology platform will focus on research and development (R&D) issues for industry and government and will result in the establishment of an EU R&D agenda. The goal of the current SENSATION program is to detect sleepiness in an actual driving situation, sensitive to chronic deprivation and health-related issues as well as time of day, and to provide this information in a meaningful way to the driver.

On May 29–30, 2006, an international conference on "Monitoring Sleep and Sleepiness—From Physiology to New Sensors" was held in Basel, Switzerland. This symposium was primarily a technical review of various projects under development for SENSATION, and it provided a forum for presenting recent advances in areas such as sensor technology, sleep physiology, and alertness prediction models and algorithms. Additional information, technical details, and research results of several promising emerging technologies and devices from this conference are presented in the following sections.

4.1 FUZZY FUSION OF PHYSIOLOGICAL INDICATORS FOR HYPOVIGILANCE-RELATED ACCIDENT PREDICTION

G. Damousis of the Centre for Research & Technology Hellas presented a fuzzy expert system for the detection of the physiological manifestations of extreme hypovigilance. The system fuses various eyelid-related features in order to provide a reliable system that both maximizes the accident prediction accuracy and generates a small number of false warnings. The system is trained to predict accidents that will occur in the next 5 minutes. For the development and testing of the system, driving simulator data from 37 subjects were used. The results of the preliminary tests show that fuzzy combination of physiological parameters presents great potential for sleep and accident prediction, while it is expected that the integration of other physiological modalities, such as EEG, will improve the performance of the system and make it suitable for commercial applications.

4.2 INDIVIDUAL DIFFERENCES IN PREDICTED DRIVING PERFORMANCE FROM SENSORY DATA AND SUBJECTIVE RATINGS

A study conducted by the Karolinska Institute was aimed at investigating individual differences in driving performance and sensory data. Data were collected from 10 subjects in a high-fidelity moving base dynamic car simulator. Subjects drove between 8:00 a.m. and 10:00 a.m. under two conditions: first, with a normal night of sleep, and then after they had worked the night shift. During the drive, eye-blink durations (BLINKD) were collected by means of electroocculogram, and driving performance was evaluated on the basis of lane drifting as measured by the standard deviation of lateral position of the vehicle (SDLAT). In addition, subjective ratings of sleepiness were collected in five-minute intervals using the Karolinska Sleepiness Scale (KSS). Accidents were scored when the vehicle went with two wheels off the right side of the road or with four wheels into the opposite lane. Data were analyzed using a generalized linear mixed model approach.

Results of the study showed that there were statistically significant relationships between KSS and BLINKD and between KSS and SDLAT. With increased sleepiness, blink durations became longer and lane drifting larger. There were also large individual differences observed for both variables independent of sleepiness levels. Subjective sleepiness, as measured by KSS, was also used to predict the probability of accidents. With increased sleepiness, the probability of an accident occurring during the subsequent five-minute segment of driving increased to approximately 10% at KSS = 9 (very sleepy, fighting sleep, effort staying awake) for an average subject. There were large individual differences in accident propensity observed with probabilities of 3% to 90% at maximum KSS. Finally, both variables BLINKD and SDLAT were found to predict accidents, and individual differences in accident propensity were larger for BLINKD than for SDLAT. The researchers concluded from their study that the probability of an accident in a driving simulator was predicted by increased subjective sleepiness, longer eye-blink durations, and increased lane drifting. However, large individual differences were also observed that must be accounted for if predictions are made for individual subjects. These individual differences were found to be largely independent of sleepiness levels and probably reflect differences in sleepiness propensity, basal physiological eye-blink processes, and driving ability.

4.3   ADVISORY SYSTEM FOR TIRED DRIVERS

Dr. Jim Horne of Loughborough University, UK gave an introductory lecture on the issues in detecting sleepiness in drivers. He then briefly discussed a new "intelligent" sleepiness warning system for drivers called the Advisory System for Tired Drivers (ASTiD). Dr. Horne stated that following fatigue-related road crashes, drivers usually deny knowledge of falling asleep at the wheel or feelings of sleepiness beforehand. This suggests they have no forewarning of sleepiness and that external aids to drowsiness detection are necessary. However, sleep does not normally occur spontaneously from an alert state. Drivers who fall asleep at the wheel have good "on-line" knowledge of sleepiness, but they underestimate the likelihood of actually falling asleep as well as the magnitude of sleepiness and its effect on impairment. Fatigued or sleepy drivers show different durations and sequences of the physiological events that precede sleep oUt. For example:

- The EEG may show neither being awake nor asleep, but a protracted state of "quasi-sleep."

- Eye closure can be delayed so that drivers are asleep with their eyes open. In fact, one in five people do not exhibit slow eyelid closures; as a result, the effectiveness of eye closure detectors is debatable.

33

- Eye blink rates are claimed to be good predictors of sleepiness, but driver blinking can be affected by factors such as outside road lighting, sunlight, oncoming headlights, in-vehicle air temperature, and state of the ventilation system.

- Reaction time is not a reliable measure of drowsiness. A study in the UK showed that the driver pushing a button on the steering wheel in respoU to a randomly generated sound from within the car gives a poor indication of driver sleepiness.

- Falling asleep can be accompanied by reduced body muscle tone (e.g., head rolling), and foot pressure on the accelerator pedal may relax. However, seat inclination can inhibit or counteract head rolling, and any vehicle decelerating depends on the dynamics of the accelerator pedal return spring in counteracting foot pressure.

Such difficulties in detecting drowsiness may not be evident in laboratory or simulator testing, since fighting sleep and fear of crashing are absent. Thus, devices must also be tested under real road and driving conditions. A key to driver sleepiness is lane drifting with cessation of steering corrections, which is the basis of the ASTiD alertness monitoring device. ASTiD both measures the predicted fatigue level using mathematical fatigue models and fatigue-related steering behavior, and provides an audible and visual warning alarm to the driver. The system uses a sleep/fatigue software model to predict levels of fatigue based on time of day, circadian clock, and the amount and quality of sleep of the operator combined with tracking of steering wheel movements. The system can be set to *require* user input (quality of prior sleep) or can be set to *assume* varying levels of default sleep quality. ASTiD has been successfully field tested in both highway and mining vehicle applications, and it is being installed in all the trucks of a leading European logistics company. Where installed, feedback from operators has been fairly positive. In general, operators felt that the system was consistent with how they were feeling, although some drivers experienced alarms when they were not feeling sleepy at all. This was observed largely when operators were not inputting their personal sleep history information.

4.4 SENSOR FOIL—CONCEPT FOR ASSESSING A DRIVER'S BODY POSTURE AND MOVEMENTS

A new sensing concept referred to as Sensor Foil (SEFO) has been developed within the SENSATION project and was described by Serge Boverie of Siemens VDO. This sensor uses a pressure-sensitive sensor foil to assess body posture and movement. The concept is based on research studies that have shown that the movements and attitudes of a human provide pertinent information to estimate wakeful and sleepy states as well as the transitions between these states. Several indicators such as body posture and movement can be used to establish a diagnostic about a person's state of wakefulness/sleepiness. The seat sensor foil design (SEFO) is a sensor matrix consisting of 64 cells (elementary sensing units). The intent of this design is to be able to measure in real time the spatial distribution of the applied pressure variation on the seat. Body movements can then be estimated with the on-line analysis algorithms. In addition, the sensor provides an estimation of body relaxation based on mechanical impedance. The system also uses an information processing and data extraction module to extract, filter, and classify the sensor output data in order to characterize the movements of the driver.

An experimental validation of the SEFO sensor was conducted to evaluate the functionality and performance of the sensor and algorithm. The sensor has been installed in an experimental vehicle, and both static and on-road driving tests have been performed. Preliminary results indicate generally good detection performance, although some misclassification problems have also been observed.

4.5 OPTALERT™—A SYSTEM FOR MONITORING EYE AND EYELID MOVEMENTS BY INFRARED REFLECTANCE OCULOGRAPHY

A research team at Sleep Diagnostics Pty Ltd in Australia, led by Dr. Murray Johns, has developed a new method called Optalert™ for monitoring the drowsiness of drivers based on the reflectance of infrared (IR) light. Brief pulses of IR light, which are invisible and safe to use, are directed at 500 Hz up at the eye from an LED positioned in a frame worn like ordinary eyeglasses. The total IR light reflected back from the eye and eyelid is measured by a phototransistor beside the LED. The ambient light measured before each pulse is subtracted from the output, which is then not affected by different environmental light levels. The output gives a measure of the position and movement of the eye and eyelid. The velocity of movement is calculated in the software as the change of position per 50 msec. For saccadic eye movements, as well as the closing and reopening of eyelids during blinks, their amplitude is very closely related to their maximum velocity. Amplitude-velocity ratios (AVRs) increase with drowsiness, as does the duration of eyelid movements and closures, whether caused by sleep deprivation or alcohol impairment. A combination of such variables has been used to create a new scale of drowsiness that has been validated against objective performance measures. The device also emits an audible alarm to warn the user of approaching drowsiness.

Optalert™ driver-drowsiness monitoring systems are currently being used by commercial vehicle operators in Australia. Despite the rather intrusive nature of the device, it reportedly has received generally positive feedback from users.

4.6 NON-INVASIVE MULTI-PARAMETER ESTIMATION OF CIRCADIAN PHASE

Alertness and sleepiness are significantly determined by an individual's sleep history and the timing of his or her circadian rhythm. For individuals performing high-vigilance tasks, such as commercial vehicle operation, monitoring and predicting the timing of circadian-induced alertness low points can provide a tool for reducing accident risk. To enable predictive capability in operational settings, however, it is necessary to measure sleep times and circadian phase timing in a non-invasive and ambulatory manner. While ambulatory actigraphy sensors can produce reasonable estimates of sleep timing, existing techniques for measuring circadian phase rely on invasive core body temperature or saliva melatonin measurements, neither of which is amenable for use outside the laboratory. There are numerous physiological measurements that exhibit circadian variations; however, no non-invasive measurements have been shown to be suitable as a stand-alone determinant of circadian phase.

Christopher Mott of the University of British Columbia presented a novel approach they are developing to circadian phase assessment using a statistical signal processing approach that combines the information from multiple non-invasive measurements into a single estimate. The technique involves a multi-parameter estimation using a Kalman filtering framework. A four-day laboratory study was performed in which a large sensor array was used to simultaneously collect non-invasive cardiac, respiratory, thermoregulatory, and motion signals. Invasive measurements of core body temperature and saliva melatonin were also collected for validation purposes. Analysis of the results confirmed that circadian components can be extracted from various non-invasive signal measurements, but that individually they are not sufficiently reliable markers. When analyzed in combination using the multi-parametric signal processing algorithm, an improved estimate of circadian phase in relation to the invasive validation measures was demonstrated. It was concluded that the multi-parametric signal processing technique makes an important step toward enabling ambulatory circadian rhythm assessment using currently available sensors and has the potential to enhance the capabilities of new ambulatory physiological sensors related to sleep and circadian rhythms.

4.7   THE IMPORTANCE OF NANOSENSORS

J. T. Devreese of the Universiteit Antwerpen (University of Antwerp) in Belgium provided a paper entitled "Sensing the Importance of Nanosensors: Feynman's Visionary 1959 Christmas Lecture." The author cites a Richard Feynman lecture in 1959 as the starting point of nanotechnology. Devreese's paper focuses on the development and implementation of nanotechnology, which underscores the primary goal of the SENSATION effort. The author discusses four reasons why nanoparticles are unique tools as sensors. First, being similar in size to many proteins, nanoparticles can operate inside cells. Second, nanosensors possess unique physical characteristics. Their sensitivity can be orders of magnitude better than that of conventional devices, and they can have fast respoU times and portability. Third, nanoparticles reveal unique physical properties that do not exist in bulk materials. And fourth, nanosensors allow for building integrated devices, providing a basis for intelligent sensors with applications for data processing, storing, and analyzing power. The paper concludes by considering prospects for the future of sensors with sizes at the nanoscale, including their usefulness as human vigilance monitoring devices. The author states that the calculated limits of sensitivity for blood pressure and pulse nanosensors, chemical and thermal nanosensors, as well as the estimated power budget for the data transfer in typical *in vivo* medical nanodevices, make them possible candidates to improve the quality of sensors for monitoring sleepiness and wakefulness.

4.8   SLEEP CONTRACTS: A PROCEDURE FOR MANAGING DAY-TO-DAY FATIGUE RISK

The Energy Institute in London, UK published a research report entitled "Viability of Using Sleep Contracts as a Control Measure in Fatigue Management" (The Energy Institute) and provided copies to attendees of the SENSATION conference. This document provides the foundation for understanding a "fatigue management system" and includes relevant tools, such as the contract itself. It is not a how-to prescription, however, and still requires expert consultation, either in-house or externally, to operationalize. This was the only discussion at the conference that centered on user and policy issues as opposed to mechanical/sensor technology. The concept of a sleep contract as an integral component in an overall fatigue management system is summarized in the following paragraphs, which are excerpted from the Energy Institute research report.

As a first step in determining the role of sleep contracts in fatigue risk management, a formal definition of the term "sleep contract" was developed. As defined by the authors, "a sleep contract is a negotiated and agreed framework for managing fatigue on a day-to-day basis that is integrated into an organization's existing Safety Management System. The framework is formally documented and makes it clear that employees and management are jointly responsible for the management of fatigue risk and states the responsibilities and accountabilities of each party." Thus, it is much more than simply a formal obligation on the part of the employee to obtain sufficient sleep prior to attending work. Nor is it merely a mechanism for management to, intentionally or unintentionally, step around fatigue risk management responsibilities.

Since a sleep contract is a new concept, it is not yet possible to provide evidence-based guidance for how best to design, implement, or operate it. Nonetheless, experience with other fatigue risk management strategies strongly indicates that for a sleep contract to be effective, the content should be agreed via a process of consultation and negotiation among employees, management, and safety professionals. The success of a sleep contract depends to a large extent on a work environment in which mutual support between employee and management exists. In this type of supportive work environment, a sleep contract is more likely to be perceived as an operational tool that has been developed to jointly assist employees and managers, rather than a disciplinary tool or a mechanism for management to avoid their responsibility regarding fatigue.

According to the Energy Institute researchers, "the theory behind a sleep contract is that, by making it a formal requirement to obtain sufficient sleep, an employee's commitment to obtaining sleep is more likely to improve. Similarly, by making it a formal requirement to report fatigue, and by providing a formal procedure for how this should be responded to, employees should be more likely to report fatigue. When an individual reports fatigue to their immediate supervisor, a sleep contract would require that both parties respond to the case in a formal, structured manner and manage the immediate and long-term risk. In this way, a sleep contract enables an organization to know its actual fatigue risk and implement the necessary controls." An additional benefit of a sleep contract is that the data collected on the incidence of fatigue can be used to track trends and to identify potential causes and countermeasures and the effectiveness of countermeasures.

For a sleep contract to be successful, its impact on key performance indicators, safety outcomes, and the behavior of individuals (employees or managers) needs to be supported, measured, and reported. For a sleep contract to be supported by the necessary operational framework it seems reasonable to recommend that it be integrated into an organization's existing Safety Management System (SMS). Within an SMS, the role of a sleep contract is twofold:

- It is a tool for monitoring fatigue and the state of contributing factors.
- It provides a negotiated framework for reporting and responding to fatigue.

Considering the potential value of sleep contracts, the authors conclude by recommending that further research be conducted to develop guidelines for the process of negotiating and implementing such a contract.

5. CONCLUSIONS

Driver drowsiness poses a major threat to highway safety, and the problem is particularly severe for commercial motor vehicle operators. Twenty-four-hour operations, high annual mileage, exposure to challenging environmental conditions, and demanding work schedules all contribute to this serious safety issue. Monitoring the driver's state of drowsiness and vigilance and providing feedback on his or her condition so that he or she can take appropriate action is one crucial step in a series of preventive measures necessary to address this problem.

This report attempts to present in a concise and summary fashion some of the scientific activities and technological approaches that are currently underway to address driver drowsiness as a critical safety issue. Several promising state-of-the-art devices and technologies were identified and evaluated against a set of proposed design guidelines. Technological advances in electronics, optics, sensory arrays, data acquisition systems, algorithm development, and machine vision have brought the goal of providing unobtrusive, real-time, affordable, 24-hour driver alertness monitoring capability much closer to reality. Considerable development effort is taking place to demonstrate the scientific validity and reliability of these technologies, but more work is required before they can be fully implemented as an integral component of an overall fatigue management program.

REFERENCES

Achermann P. 2004. The two-process model of sleep regulation revisited. *Aviation, Space, and Environmental Medicine* 75(3):Section II.

Aguirre A, Croke D, Guttkuhn R, Heitmann A, Moore-Ede M, Trutschel U. 2004. Circadian alertness simulator for fatigue risk assessment in transportation: Application to reduce frequency and severity of truck accidents. *Aviation, Space, and Environmental Medicine* 75(3):Section II.

Akerstedt T, Folkard S, Portin C. 2004. Predictions from the three-process model of alertness. *Aviation, Space, and Environmental Medicine* 75(3):Section II.

Balkin TJ, Belenky G, Eddy DR, Hursh SR, Miller JC, Redmond DP, Storm WF, Thorne DR. 2004. Fatigue models for applied research in warfighting. *Aviation, Space, and Environmental Medicine* 75(3):Section II.

Barr L, Hitz J, Popkin S, Wilson B. 2002. Detailed plan for an independent evaluation of a drowsy driver warning system. Cambridge, MA: Volpe National Transportation Systems Center, National Highway Transportation Safety Administration, U.S. Dept. of Transportation. Project Memorandum DOT-VNTSC-HW11Q-PM-01-42.

Bekiaris E, Nikolaou S, Mousadakou A. 2004a. Design guidelines for driver drowsiness detection and avoidance [online report]. System for effective Assessment of driver vigilance and Warning According to traffic risK Estimation (AWAKE) Deliverable 9.1 [cited 1 Nov 2006]. Thessaloniki, Greece: European Commission, Information Society Technologies, AWAKE Consortium. Available online: www.awake-eu.org/pdf/d9_1.pdf.

Bekiaris E, Dunne S, Nikolaou S, Ruffini G. Information Society Technologies (IST) Programme: SENSATION. 2004b. Project presentation. Deliverable No. D5.1.3.

Belyavin AJ, Spencer MB. 2004 Modeling performance and alertness: The QinetiQ approach. *Aviation, Space, and Environmental Medicine* 75(3):Section II.

Bierman DM, Byrne VE, Carnahan B, Davis RK, France E, Grace R, Gricourt D, Legrand J-M, Staszewski JJ. 1999. A drowsy driver detection system for heavy vehicles. Proceedings of the Ocular Measures of Driver Alertness Conference, April 26–27, in Herndon, VA.

Borbely A. 1982. A. A two-process model of sleep regulation. *Human Neurobiology* 1:195–204.

Boyle LN, Najm WG, Stearns MD. 2001. Detailed plan for an independent evaluation of the automotive collision avoidance system field operational test. Cambridge, MA: Volpe National Transportation Systems Center, National Highway Transportation Safety Administration, U.S. Department of Transportation. Project Memorandum DOT-VMTSC-HS116-PM-01-09.

Cleveland D. 1999. Unobtrusive eyelid closure and visual point of regard measurement system. Proceedings of the Ocular Measures of Driver Alertness Conference, April 26–27, in Herndon, VA.

Dawson D, Fletcher A, Roach GD. 2004. Model to predict work-related fatigue based on hours of work. *Aviation, Space, and Environmental Medicine* 75(3):Section II.

Dinges DF, Mallis MM. 1998. Managing fatigue by drowsiness detection: Can technological promises be realised? Proceedings of the 3rd Fatigue in Transportation Conference: Managing Fatigue in Transportation. Fremantle, Western Australia. Reprinted in *Managing Fatigue in Transportation,* Hartley LR (ed.). Bingley, UK: Emerald Group Publishing Limited: pp. 209-30.

Dinges DF, Mallis MM, Mejdal S, Nguyen TT. 2004. Summary of the key features of seven biomathematical models of human fatigue and performance. Aviation, Space, and Environmental Medicine 75(3):Section II.

Dinges DF. 1997. The promise and challenges of technologies for monitoring operator vigilance. Proceedings of the International Conference on Managing Fatigue in Transportation, American Trucking Associations Foundation, April 29–30, in Tampa Florida.

Eddy DR, Hursh SR. 2001. Fatigue avoidance scheduling tool (FAST). Brooks Air Force Base, TX: US Air Force Research Laboratory. Report No. AFRL-HE-BR-TR-2001-0140.

Energy Institute. 2006. Viability of using sleep contracts as a control measure in fatigue management [report online]. London, England: Energy Institute [cited 1 Nov 2006]. Available online: www.energyinst.org.uk/content/files/iprfatigue.pdf.

Eskandarian A, Sayed R. 2005. Driving simulator experiment: Detecting driver fatigue by monitoring eye and steering activity [online presentation]. National DefeU Industrial Association 3rd Annual Intelligent Vehicle Systems Symposium, June 9–12, in Traverse City, MI [cited 1 Nov 2006]. Available online: proceedings.ndia.org/3570/session5/Eskandarian.ppt.

Liu X, Xu F, Fujimura K. 2002. Real-time eye detection and tracking for driver observation under various light conditions. Paper presented at the Intelligent Vehicle Symposium, IEEE. 2:344-51 [cited 1 Nov 2006]. Available online: ieeexplore.ieee.org/Xplore/login.jsp?url=/stamp/stamp.jsp?arnumber=1187975&isnumber=26633.

Grace R. 2006. Drowsy driver monitor and warning system [online paper]. Pittsburgh, PA: Robotics Institute, Carnegie Mellon University [cited 1 Nov 2006]. Available online: www.attentiontechnology.com/docs/DrowsyDriverMonitor.pdf.

Hartley L, Horberry T, Mabbott N, Krueger GP. 2000. Review of fatigue detection and prediction technologies [working paper online]. Melbourne, Victoria, Australia: National Road Transport Commission [cited 1 Nov 2006]. ISBN: 0-642-54469-7. Available online: www.ntc.gov.au/filemedia/Reports/ReviewFatigueDetectionandPredict.pdf

Ji Q, Lan P, Zhu Z. 2004. Real-time nonintrusive monitoring and prediction of driver fatigue. IEEE Transactions on Vehicular Technology 53(4).

Ji Q, Lan P, Looney C. 2006. A probabilistic framework for modeling and real-time monitoring human fatigue [paper online]. Troy, NY: Electrical, Computer, and Systems Engineering Department; Rensselaer Polytechnic Institute [cited 1 Nov 2006]. Available online: www.ecse.rpi.edu/~qji/Fatigue/sY_paper.pdf.

Ji Q, Yang X. 2002. Real-time eye, gaze, and face pose tracking for monitoring driver vigilance. *Real-Time Imaging* 8:357–77.

Johns Hopkins University Applied Physics Laboratory. 2006. Microwave and acoustic detection of drowsiness [report online]. Laurel, MD: The Johns Hopkins University Applied Physics Laboratory [cited 1 Nov 2006]. Available online: www.jhuapl.edu/ott/technologies/technology/articles/P01471.asp.

Krueger GP. 2004. Technologies and methods for monitoring driver alertness and detecting driver fatigue: A review applicable to long haul truck driving. Arlington, VA: American Transportation Research Institute.

National Highway Traffic Safety Administration (NHTSA). 1997. Report to Congress on the National Highway Traffic Safety Administration ITS program, program progress during 1992–1996 and strategic plan for 1997–2002. ITS Joint Program Office, U.S. Department of Transportation: Washington, DC.

Rosekind MR. 1998. Managing fatigue in transportation: No magic bullet. Hearing on fatigue and its safety effects on the commercial motor vehicle and railroad industries. United States Senate, Committee on Commerce, Science and Transportation.

Sayed R, Eskandarian A, Oskard M. 2001. Driver drowsiness detection using artificial neural networks. Paper presented at the National Research Council (US), 80th annual meeting of the Transportation Research Board, January 2001 in Washington, DC. Paper No. 01-2113.

Sullivan JJ. 2003. Fighting fatigue [article online]. *Public Roads* 67(2) [cited 1 Nov 2006]. Available online: www.tfhrc.gov/pubrds/03sep/04.htm

Whitlock A. 2002. Driver vigilance devices: Systems review [paper online]. Farnham, Surrey, United Kingdom: Quintec Associates Limited [cited 1 Nov 2006]. Available online: www.rssb.co.uk/pdf/reports/Research/T024%20Driver%20vigilance%20devices%20-%20systems%20review.pdf.

Wierwille WW. 1999. Desired attributes of drowsy driver monitoring and candidate technologies for implementation. Proceedings of the Ocular Measures of Driver Alertness Conference, April 26–27, in Herndon, VA.

www.ingramcontent.com/pod-product-compliance
Lightning Source LLC
Chambersburg PA
CBHW080446290526
45791CB00008BA/2628